MAKING SENSE of
Clinical Teaching

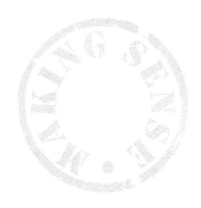

MAKING SENSE of

Clinical Teaching

Edited by
Samy A Azer

MD, PhD (USyd), MEd (UNSW) FACG, MPH (UNSW)
Professor of Medical Education and Chair of Curriculum Development &
Research Unit, College of Medicine, King Saud University, Saudi Arabia
Formerly Professor of Medical Education and Chair of Medical Education Research &
Development Unit, Faculty of Medicine, Universiti Teknologi MARA, Malaysia
Visiting Professor of Medical Education, Faculty of Medicine, University of Toyama, Japan
Director of the Australian Professional Teaching (APT), Melbourne, Australia
Formerly Senior Lecturer in Medical Education, Faculty of Medicine, Dentistry and
Health Sciences, University of Melbourne and University of Sydney, Australia
Associate Editor *BMC Medical Education*, United Kingdom

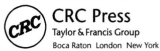

CRC Press
Taylor & Francis Group
Boca Raton London New York

CRC Press is an imprint of the
Taylor & Francis Group, an **informa** business

CRC Press
Taylor & Francis Group
6000 Broken Sound Parkway NW, Suite 300
Boca Raton, FL 33487-2742

© 2013 by Taylor & Francis Group, LLC
CRC Press is an imprint of Taylor & Francis Group, an Informa business

No claim to original U.S. Government works

Printed on acid-free paper by CPI Group (UK) Ltd, Croydon
Version Date: 20130125

International Standard Book Number-13: 978-1-4441-4412-3 (Paperback)

Library of Congress Cataloging-in-Publication Data

Making sense of clinical teaching : a hands-on guide to success / editor, Samy Azer.
    p. ; cm. -- (Making sense)
  Includes bibliographical references and index.
  ISBN 978-1-4441-4412-3 (pbk. : alk. paper)
  I. Azer, Samy A. II. Series: Making sense (Boca Raton, Fla.)
  [DNLM: 1. Education, Medical--methods. 2. Teaching--methods. 3. Education, Medical--organization & administration. 4. Problem-Based Learning. W 18]

R735
610.71--dc23   2013001643

Visit the Taylor & Francis Web site at
http://www.taylorandfrancis.com

and the CRC Press Web site at
http://www.crcpress.com

Dedication

To my teachers and mentors
who motivated me and opened many doors during my career

To my students in Australia, Japan, Malaysia and Saudi Arabia who
became colleagues

To my family, and my daughters Sarah and Diana
for your love and support

In memory of my parents
for your unconditional love and encouragement

Contents

Contributors

Ayman A Abdo MD FACP

Associate Professor of Medicine, Consultant Hepatologist, Director, KSU Liver Disease Research Center, Vice Dean for Quality and Development, College of Medicine, King Saud University, Riyadh, Saudi Arabia

Hamza M Abdulghani FRCGP MMED

Associate Professor of Medical Education, and Chair of Assessment & Evaluation Unit, College of Medicine, King Saud University, Riyadh, Saudi Arabia

Mubarak bin Fahad Al-Faran MD

Dean of College of Medicine and Professor of Ophthalmology, King Saud University, Riyadh, Saudi Arabia

Fawaz Al-hussain MBBS FRCPC MPH

Assistant Professor of Neurology, Consultant Neurologist, College of Medicine, King Saud University, Riyadh, Saudi Arabia

Sami Al-Nassar MD FRCSC

Assistant Professor of Surgery, Consultant Thoracic Surgeon, Chairman, Department of Medical Education, Head, Division of Thoracic Surgery, College of Medicine, King Saud University, Riyadh, Saudi Arabia

Badran Alomar PHD

Professor and President, King Saud University, Riyadh, Saudi Arabia

Muslim M Al-Saadi MD FCCP

Professor of Paediatrics and Vice Dean for Academic Affairs, College of Medicine, King Saud University, Riyadh, Saudi Arabia

Mohammad Y Al-Shehri MD FACS

Vice Rector for Health Sciences and Professor of Surgery, King Saud University, Riyadh, Saudi Arabia

Zubair Amin MD MHPE

Associate Professor, Department of Paediatrics, Yong Loo Lin School of Medicine National University of Singapore, Singapore

Samy A Azer MD PHD

Professor of Medical Education and Chair of Curriculum Development and Research Unit, College of Medicine, King Saud University, Saudi Arabia; formerly Professor of Medical Education and Chair of Medical Education Research and Development Unit, Faculty of Medicine, Universiti Teknologi MARA, Malaysia; Visiting Professor of Medical Education, Faculty of Medicine, University of Toyama, Japan; Director of Australian Professional Teaching (APT), Melbourne, Australia; formerly Senior Lecturer in Medical Education, Faculty of Medicine, Dentistry and Health Sciences, University of Melbourne and University of Sydney, Australia; Associate Editor *BMC Medical Education*, United Kingdom

Nervana Bayoumy MD PHD

Assistant Professor of Physiology, Consultant Molecular Biologist, Director of Academic Quality Unit, College of Medicine, King Saud University, Riyadh, Saudi Arabia

Saad Bindawas PHD

Physical Therapy Assistant Professor, College of Applied Medical Sciences, King Saud University, Riyadh, Saudi Arabia

Engle Angela Chan PHD

Associate Professor, Associate Head (Pre-service Education), School of Nursing, The Hong Kong Polytechnic University, Hong Kong

Peter Dieter PHD

Professor of Biochemistry, Medical School Representative for International Relations, Dresden University of Technology, Faculty of Medicine Carl Gustav Carus, Institute of Physiological Chemistry, Dresden, Germany

Denise M Dupras MD PHD

Professor of Medicine, Division of Primary Care Internal Medicine, College of Medicine, Mayo Clinic, Rochester, Minnesota, USA

Gudrun Edgren PHD

Associate Professor of Medical Education, Director of Centre for Teaching and Learning, Faculty of Medicine, Lund University, Lund, Sweden

Anthony PS Guerrero MD

Professor of Psychiatry and Clinical Professor of Pediatrics, Department of Psychiatry, John A. Burns School of Medicine, University of Hawaii, Honolulu, Hawaii, USA

Rana Hassanato MD

Consultant in Clinical Biochemistry and Chair of Biochemistry Unit, College of Medicine, King Saud University, Riyadh, Saudi Arabia

Susan J Hawken MBChB Dip Obs FRNZCGP MHSc(Hons)

Senior Lecturer, Department of Psychological Medicine, Faculty of Medical and Health Sciences, University of Auckland, Auckland, New Zealand

Marcus A Henning PHD

Senior Lecturer, Centre for Medical and Health Sciences Education, Faculty of Medical and Health Sciences, University of Auckland, Auckland, New Zealand

Onishi Hirotaka MD

Assistant Professor of Medical Education, International Research Center for Medical Education, University of Tokyo, Japan

Kun-Long Hung MD PHD

Professor and Associate Dean, Fu-Jen Catholic University, New Taipei, Taiwan

Richard Kasuya MD

Associate Dean for Medical Education and Professor of Medicine at the John A. Burns School of Medicine, University of Hawaii; Honolulu, Hawaii, USA

Tadahiko Kozu MD

Professor Emeritus, Tokyo Women's Medical University Councillor, Japan Medical Education Foundation, Tokyo, Japan

Chi-Wan Lai MD

Chairman, Taiwan Medical Accreditation Council, and Chair Professor, AHT Medical Education Promotion Foundation, Taiwan

Cindy LK Lam MD

Danny DP Ho Professor in Family Medicine, Department of Family Medicine and Primary Care, Li Ka Shing Faculty of Medicine, the University of Hong Kong, Hong Kong SAR, China

Sam Leinster MD

Emeritus Professor and former Dean of the University of East Anglia School of Medicine, UK

Michelle McLean PHD, MEd

Academic Lead, PBL and Small Group Teaching, Faculty of Health Sciences and Medicine, Bond University, Queensland, Australia

Jill SM Omori MD

Director of Predoctoral Education, Department of Family Medicine and Community Health, John A. Burns School of Medicine, University of Hawaii, Honolulu, Hawaii, USA

Ray Peterson PHD

Associate Professor in Education, Faculty of Health Sciences, University of Adelaide, Australia

Julie Quinlivan MD PHD

Pro Vice Chancellor and Executive Dean of Medicine. University of Notre Dame, Sydney, Australia

Subha Ramani MD MPH

Associate Professor of Medicine, Boston University School of Medicine, Boston, Massachusetts, USA

Damon H Sakai MD

Associate Professor of Medicine, Director of Medical Student Education, and Director of the Office of Medical Education, John A. Burns School of Medicine, University of Hawaii, Honolulu, Hawaii, USA

Patricia S Sexton DHEd

Associate Dean for Curriculum, Associate Professor of Family Medicine, Kirksville College of Osteopathic Medicine, Kirksville, Missouri, USA

Roger Strasser MD

Dean and CEO, Professor of Rural Health, Northern Ontario School of Medicine, Laurentian and Lakehead Universities, Northern Ontario, Canada

Masami Tagawa MD PHD MHPE

Professor of Medical Education and Director, Center for Innovation in Medical and Dental Education, Kagoshima University Graduate School of Medical and Dental Sciences, Sakuragaoka, Kagoshima, Japan

Margareta Troein MD PHD

Professor, General Practitioner, Department of Clinical Sciences Malmö, Faculty of Medicine, Lund University, Lund, Sweden

Allyn Walsh MD CCFP

Chair of Student Affairs and Professor of Family Medicine in Michael G DeGroote School of Medicine, McMaster University, Hamilton, Ontario, Canada

Ian Wilson MD PHD

Professor of Medical Education and Chair of Medical Education Unit, School of Medicine, University of Western Sydney, Sydney, New South Wales, Australia

Yi-Chu Yang MD MS

Chairman, Department of Community Medicine, Cathay General Hospital, Taipei, Taiwan

Foreword

The introduction of integrated and student-centred curricula to health professional programmes has revolutionized how health professional teachers conduct their teaching sessions. Clinical teachers currently require a range of skills, qualities and professional attitudes in order to help their students to develop their skills and get the best out of their clinical sessions. Evidence shows that students learn to develop their professional attitudes and skills not through lectures about professionalism or small group discussion but rather from observation of their teachers as they interact with them, examine patients and work on their problems, as well as from teachers' interactions with other members in the professional health team. For students, teachers are their role models and a wide range of skills are learnt on a day-to-day basis by mimicking the actions of their teachers. Therefore, clinical teachers need to be prepared to teach students *how* to learn, not only what to learn, and turn challenges into learning opportunities. Although novice clinical teachers will need mentors and continuous feedback to help them develop their teaching skills, there is definitely a need for resources to guide them in this process. However, there are few resources available covering these needs.

This book provides readers with the opportunity to interact with 60 clinical scenarios that mimic real teaching/learning situations and enables them to analyse the situation, think about possible contributing causes, generate hypotheses, look at related best evidence, develop an action plan and reflect on take-home messages and lessons learnt. The references at the end of each subchapter provide useful resources for readers interested in further information.

We are pleased that Professor Samy Azer, the editor of this book, currently a member of King Saud University, has used his skills in clinical medicine, research and clinical education to provide clinical teachers with an invaluable resource.

It is a pleasure to recommend this book to you. Despite the small size of the book, it comprises 60 subchapters written by 39 contributors from 13 countries which add to the value of the book. This book will be useful to novice clinical teachers, small group tutors, clinical teachers who are willing to further their skills, and clinical deans, as well as chairs of medical education departments/units. It highly deserves a place on each clinical teacher's desk.

Professor Badran Alomar
President of King Saud University
Riyadh, Saudi Arabia

Preface

With the recent adoption of student-centred learning approaches, clinical teachers are no longer transmitters of factual knowledge or 'spoon feeders'. Teachers' responsibilities in current education are now widely varied and include encouraging critical thinking, fostering curiosity and searching for explanations, monitoring group progress, facilitating students' collaborative learning, giving constructive feedback and motivating students to achieve their potential.

Making Sense of Clinical Teaching is written for teachers who want to reach their potential and achieve excellence in their profession. The contents of this book are the result of several years of extensive research in this area and reflect the editor's experiences in teaching and training staff in higher education. They also reflect the views 39 medical and health professionals from a number of countries including Australia, New Zealand, Japan, Hong Kong, Singapore, Taiwan, Saudi Arabia, United Kingdom, Sweden, United States and Canada.

Over the last ten years, I have run more than 70 workshops to enhance the teaching and facilitation skills of teachers and educators. These workshops were conducted for academic staff and clinicians from several universities in Australia, South East Asia, and beyond. In these workshops, I ask the participants to write down the name of the best teacher they have ever had and list what was unique about this teacher. In what way was he or she different? What qualities did he or she possess?

Interestingly, certain qualities are common among many of these teachers. Even when I asked secondary and primary school teachers in Australia to provide me with their views, there were no differences between the three groups. Great teachers share these qualities regardless of the subject they teach, their academic background or the level of the students they teach.

The design of this book encourages teachers to identify the good qualities they have, to learn how they can improve their potential, influence and develop other teachers around them, and leave a mark on their journey to success.

Making Sense of Clinical Teaching is a package that will enable you to:

- Add new skills to your teaching expertise
- Stimulate your creative thinking
- Challenge your current teaching and provide you with the tools to reach your potential
- Meet the needs of your students in a win–win approach
- Construct new strategies in your department/schools
- Mentor your teaching and learning skills.

Making Sense of Clinical Teaching provides you with:

- 60 case scenarios discussed in 60 subchapters
- Case discussions and key questions that can broaden the concept discussed and help you identify key principles
- Action plans related to the case scenario and management options
- Recent research outcomes in this area
- Take-home messages
- Resources for further reading.

Making Sense of Clinical Teaching is a book that you will turn to again and again for nourishment on your teaching journey and will help you develop your own leadership in teaching and learning. I am interested in receiving your comments and feedback.

Professor Samy A Azer
Professor of Medical Education
Chair of Medical Education and Research Unit
King Saud University
Azer2000@optusnet.com.au

Acknowledgements

I would like to thank my students in Australia, Japan, Malaysia and Saudi Arabia for their valuable comments and suggestions during the different stages of writing this book. I also thank the publisher's staff for their help and support throughout the process, particularly Joanna Koster, publisher; Stephen Clausard, Susie Bond, Holly Regan-Jones and Joanna Walker for their help and support during the process of communication with the subchapters' contributors, project editing, and the proofreading of the manuscript. I also thank Amina Dudhia for the book cover design.

I would like to thank the reviewers of the early submission of the book proposal for their comments and valuable suggestions. I thank Diana Azer for her help with the revision of the whole manuscript and her valuable suggestions throughout the process of creating this book.

Finally, I would like to thank Professor Badran Alomar, the President of King Saud University, for his encouragement and support and for writing the Foreword of the book.

Introduction

Samy A Azer

CLINICAL TEACHER

Clinical teachers, as is the case with other university teachers, are described as scholars as they are able to advance or transform knowledge through application of their intellects in an informed, disciplined and creative manner.[1] This requires the creation of new knowledge and its dissemination through peer review and publication. Therefore, the pursuit of scholarship should target development, implementation and the documentation of a lifelong learning journey, and the use of evidence-based information and reflection on teaching.[2] The evaluation of teachers' knowledge and approaches to lifelong learning can be assessed by peer review and constructive feedback. In addition, the use of a teaching portfolio is a key source of information which can provide a valid tool to assess faculty members' scholarly approach and development in teaching and learning.[3]

In other words, research, teaching and services (to the schools, university and wider community) are fundamental activities of academic life and represent scholarship in medical and health professions education.[4] Among these activities, the creation of new knowledge and its dissemination to the wider academic and research community through peer review and publication are crucial. Other activities include management, administration and leadership in the educational systems in the medical and health professions, as well as ensuring successful implementation of changes that can benefit students, health services, quality of care and the profession.

Considering the fact that the environment for research work is explicit and well-developed in academia, there is a need for such an environment for the development of scholarship education. For example, there is a well-developed culture for training and collaboration in research work, competition for grants and presentation of research outcomes to peers. Academics belong to professional societies, attend national meetings, publish in peer-reviewed journals and participate freely in providing services to the profession. This includes volunteering to become a peer reviewer, contributing to professional societies' activities and undertaking leadership professional responsibilities. In almost all universities, there is strong emphasis on research outcomes, publications in peer-reviewed journals and acquiring grants obtained by academics as essential prerequisites for promotion and rewards.

The same applies to clinical practise in medical and allied health professions. For example, there are clear, well-defined standards in patient care, professional conduct, expectations and clinical practises. There are also well-established training programmes and examinations in order for junior clinicians to progress to specialist/consultant positions in a particular area in clinical practise. Academic status and positions are a function of expertise, input to clinical research and performance within a specialty. Therefore, progression of an academic career for a clinician is based on patient care and clinical research, not education and teaching undergraduate students.[5] Clinical teachers usually agree to contribute to students' education because they enjoy teaching and believe that students will be their residents in a few years to come. However, most clinicians do not believe that teaching is their priority. Compared to patient care and clinical research, they themselves did not receive formal training in teaching or assessment of learners, and may feel that teaching takes a great deal of their time.[6] Some clinical teachers believe that they have been teaching students for a good number of years, and they are not in need of guidance or monitoring by medical/health education departments.[7,8] This belief may lead them to reject changes in the curriculum and resist collaboration with medical/health education departments. Heads of clinical departments often fail to distinguish between teaching as a scholarly activity and teaching as a routine service.

These conditions and such beliefs are not limited to a particular discipline or a particular country. On the contrary, they represent a common challenge to scholarship in education in top universities, as well as in universities with average/low-ranking status, although the degree of challenge or understanding of what makes scholarship education may vary.

SCHOLARSHIP IN EDUCATION

In 1990, Boyer proposed a four-part concept of scholarship that comprised the application, integration, teaching and discovery of new knowledge.[9] However, the four components proposed by Boyer did not provide a clear understanding as to how a scholar in education is different from excellent teaching and this suggests that there are other key components not highlighted in Boyer's model. Nine years later, Hutchings and Shulman[8] added new dimensions to the definition and highlighted that scholarship in education occurs when it is public, open to evaluation, transparent and has been presented in such a way that allows for other academics to build on it further and explores students' learning.

In recognition of the challenges in medical and health professional curricula, there has been an increase in the number of diploma and Master's-level degrees in medical/health education. Also an increasing number of fellowships have been created, purely dedicated to medical/ health professional education.[10,11] Although there is a general belief that the completion of such degrees is important for staff development, there is no evidence that successful completion of such degrees on their own will guarantee that graduates become scholars in medical/ health education. In fact, the work of Goldszmidt et al.[12] shows that encouraging faculty to participate in education scholarships should not be limited only to those with advanced degrees nor rely on having a degree in medical education as a prerequisite for such training. In my experience, there are a good number of faculty members in different colleges who have completed diplomas or Master's in medical/health education but were unable to translate the knowledge and skills gained during their studies to create innovative ideas in teaching and learning, help in the advancement of knowledge and skills in their area of expertise, or demonstrate leadership in medical/health education. Such observations have also been highlighted by other researchers.[11,12] This means that scholarship in education is not necessarily dependent on completing a degree in medical/health education. Rather, it is about the desire of teachers to continuously work beyond the goal of completing a degree and remain committed to lifelong effective achievement comprising a number of activities reflecting scholarship in education.

Glassick et al.[13,14] proposed six common criteria for the assessment of scholarship in education: clear goals, adequate preparation, appropriate methods, significant results, effective communication and reflective critique. In other words, scholarship in education includes creating material for new curriculum, introducing innovative teaching and learning approaches, creating a web-based educational site, enhancing staff and students' skills in attending training programmes, as well as writing textbooks or other educational publications that attract peer review and critical evaluation before publication. Such academic activities together with reflective critique, lifelong learning and adding new dimensions to the discipline and/or profession represent strong examples of scholarship in education.[15–18]

HOW IS SCHOLARSHIP DIFFERENT FROM EXCELLENCE IN TEACHING?

Scholarship in education is neither about completing a degree in medical/health education[12] nor about demonstrating excellence in teaching. Scholarship in education is a continuum of achievements rather than merely delivering successful teaching sessions. Scholarly teaching has to be public, susceptible to critical review, and accessible for exchange and use for other scholars.[12,19] Defining rewards and criteria for rewarding scholarly teachers should be given a priority. The vice-chanceries, deans, committee of deans, professional bodies, academic centres, and educational organizations have vital roles in promoting educational scholarship.

Over the last 20 years, several changes have been introduced to medical curricula and a wide range of teaching/learning options, such as integrated teaching, small group tutorials, problem-based learning, team-based learning, core curriculum with electives or options, and student-led seminars, have been advocated. These changes emphasize student-centred learning, self-directed learning, and development of students' knowledge, skills and competencies in areas learnt. The use of e-learning and learning technology has supported these changes and prepared students to move from teacher-centred curricula to student-centred learning. These changes may be seen as a loss of teachers' control, a move that devalues the role of teachers, and raises doubts about the impact of these changes on students' learning outcomes. On the contrary, the new curricula necessitate a significant input by teachers to develop the integrated curriculum design, create the material needed for students' learning, and introduce changes to the assessment. In other words, the changes in the curriculum do not only aim at enhancing students' learning, but also developing teachers' skills in a way that ensures achieving optimum outcomes. The changes in the curriculum also aim at the development of the profession and medical education research, as well as the enhancement of the teacher's skills and providing opportunities to teachers to demonstrate excellence in teaching and, through a continuum of achievements, to become scholarly teachers.

Challenges facing clinical and academic teachers

- Clinical teachers are new to evidence-based teaching and the need for continuous training in areas such as facilitation skills, use of simulation in teaching, and how to teach knowledge, skills and professional attitude in one setting is imperative.[20,21]

- Evaluation of clinical teaching for the individual teacher and for clinical programmes is lacking and there are no clearly defined standards that can be implemented. This lack of definition in many situations can lead to a feeling that long teaching experience and/ or the completion of a degree in education are adequate for the entitlement of the title of scholar in education.[22,23]

- There is limited or no funding available for clinical teaching research. This applies to governmental bodies and university grants.[6]

- Many academic teachers begin their life as clinicians or basic science academics who then move to a professional career in education that may focus mainly on research, teaching, management, administration or more than one of these domains. These educators may be employed by universities, teaching hospitals, education centres or colleges. These differences in background, the nature of their professional career in education and their employers may create a challenge regarding the definition of a scholar in education.[4,19]

- While clinical care and research generate income for medical and health profession schools, education in these schools costs money and the deans have to work hard to allocate funds for education.

- Clinicians and academics commit most of their time to patient and health care, as well as their research. They find it difficult to strike a balance between these priorities and teaching. So the challenge is to reconsider the role and place of teaching in medical and health-care professions.

REACHING YOUR POTENTIAL AS A CLINICAL TEACHER

Think about a clinical teacher with whom you were a student. He or she does not have to be the teacher you liked least, but should be the teacher with whom you had the most difficulty in achieving learning and developing your skills. Describe this teacher.

Focuses on students' needs	8	7	6	5	4	3	2	1	Doesn't focus on students' needs
Works with passion	8	7	6	5	4	3	2	1	Works with no passion
Upholds the professional values	8	7	6	5	4	3	2	1	Doesn't abide by professional values
Enthusiastic about clinical teaching	8	7	6	5	4	3	2	1	Not enthusiastic about clinical teaching
Creates a climate of trust	8	7	6	5	4	3	2	1	Creates unhealthy environment
Encourages students to learn from mistakes	8	7	6	5	4	3	2	1	Doesn't encourage students
Help students to redefine failure	8	7	6	5	4	3	2	1	Doesn't help students
Accepts uncertainty in medicine	8	7	6	5	4	3	2	1	Doesn't accept uncertainty in medicine
Accessible/available to students	8	7	6	5	4	3	2	1	Not available to students
Communicates effectively	8	7	6	5	4	3	2	1	Communicates poorly
Encourages input from others	8	7	6	5	4	3	2	1	Doesn't encourage input from others
Acts with integrity	8	7	6	5	4	3	2	1	Has no integrity
Provides a model of professional ethics	8	7	6	5	4	3	2	1	Doesn't show professional ethics
Shows a caring attitude	8	7	6	5	4	3	2	1	No caring attitude
Motivates students	8	7	6	5	4	3	2	1	Demotivates students
Monitors student progress	8	7	6	5	4	3	2	1	Doesn't monitor progress

Motivates co-workers	8	7	6	5	4	3	2	1 Demotivates co-workers
A good sense of humour	8	7	6	5	4	3	2	1 No sense of humour
Doesn't speak negatively	8	7	6	5	4	3	2	1 Speaks negatively
Encourages diversity	8	7	6	5	4	3	2	1 Against diversity
Respects people of diverse background	8	7	6	5	4	3	2	1 Doesn't respect people of diverse background
Enforces equal opportunities	8	7	6	5	4	3	2	1 Doesn't enforce equal opportunities
Maintains positive relationships with students	8	7	6	5	4	3	2	1 Poor relationships
Uses a wide range of teaching approaches	8	7	6	5	4	3	2	1 Uses one approach
Stimulates higher-order thinking skills	8	7	6	5	4	3	2	1 Focuses on memorization
Presents difficult concepts comprehensibly	8	7	6	5	4	3	2	1 Doesn't present difficult concepts comprehensibly
Encourages evidence to a critique	8	7	6	5	4	3	2	1 Doesn't encourage evidence to a critique
Teaches memorably	8	7	6	5	4	3	2	1 Doesn't teach memorably
Models a close doctor–patient relationship	8	7	6	5	4	3	2	1 Doesn't model a close doctor–patient relationship
Uses education in community development	8	7	6	5	4	3	2	1 Doesn't use education in community development
Teaches students how to think	8	7	6	5	4	3	2	1 Teaches what to think
Explores with probing questions	8	7	6	5	4	3	2	1 Doesn't explore with probing questions
Discusses ideas in an organized way	8	7	6	5	4	3	2	1 Doesn't discuss ideas in an organized way
Helps students focus on key issues	8	7	6	5	4	3	2	1 Doesn't help students focus on key issues

Trains students to think strategically	8	7	6	5	4	3	2	1	Doesn't train students to think strategically
Motivates students to create new ideas	8	7	6	5	4	3	2	1	Doesn't motivate students to create new ideas
Fosters innovations	8	7	6	5	4	3	2	1	Doesn't foster innovations
Shows enthusiasm for creative ideas	8	7	6	5	4	3	2	1	Doesn't show enthusiasm for creative ideas
Encourages students to work in groups	8	7	6	5	4	3	2	1	Doesn't encourage students to work in groups
Encourages collaborative learning	8	7	6	5	4	3	2	1	Doesn't encourage collaborative learning
Encourages links in education	8	7	6	5	4	3	2	1	Doesn't encourage links in education
Listens to discover students' educational needs	8	7	6	5	4	3	2	1	Doesn't listen to discover students' educational needs
Values students	8	7	6	5	4	3	2	1	Doesn't value students
Provides constructive feedback	8	7	6	5	4	3	2	1	Doesn't provide constructive feedback
Supports students to grow	8	7	6	5	4	3	2	1	Doesn't support students to grow
Teaches students how to monitor their progress	8	7	6	5	4	3	2	1	Doesn't teach students how to monitor their progress
Seeks to learn and incorporate new skills	8	7	6	5	4	3	2	1	Doesn't seek to learn and incorporate new skills
Seeks feedback	8	7	6	5	4	3	2	1	Doesn't seek feedback
Keeps up-to-date	8	7	6	5	4	3	2	1	Doesn't keep up to date
Uses technology to facilitate teaching and learning	8	7	6	5	4	3	2	1	Doesn't use technology to facilitate teaching and learning
Monitors his/her progress	8	7	6	5	4	3	2	1	Doesn't monitor his/her progress

Contributes to course design	8	7	6	5	4	3	2	1	Doesn't contribute to course design
Contributes to publication on education	8	7	6	5	4	3	2	1	Doesn't contribute to publication on education
Demonstrates self-development	8	7	6	5	4	3	2	1	Doesn't demonstrate self-development
Demonstrates creativity in teaching strategies	8	7	6	5	4	3	2	1	Doesn't demonstrate creativity in teaching strategies
Committed to professional development	8	7	6	5	4	3	2	1	Is not committed to professional development
Shares in managing changes in the curriculum	8	7	6	5	4	3	2	1	Doesn't share in managing changes in the curriculum
Uses evidence-based teaching	8	7	6	5	4	3	2	1	Doesn't use evidence-based teaching
Contributes to research in clinical education	8	7	6	5	4	3	2	1	Doesn't contribute to research in clinical education
Encourages students to undertake research and publish their work	8	7	6	5	4	3	2	1	Doesn't encourage students to undertake research and publish their work

Use this list again to assess yourself. How do you see your role as a teacher? Make a copy of the list, reflect on each item and give yourself a score of how you see yourself from a score of 1 to 8. You could also ask a colleague and your students to use this list in scoring you and providing you with feedback on your role as a teacher. Such assessment will provide you with a wealth of knowledge about your role as a teacher, areas you are excelling in and areas that need further improvement.

Identify any obstacles that are holding you back and develop an action plan by which you could improve your skills in a particular area. Read the chapters related to particular areas and amend your action plan in light of the knowledge you have gained. Work on implementing your plan. You may also read resources provided at the end of each subchapter and use knowledge provided to enhance your skills in improving your performance.

Reflect on your day-to-day teaching practises and your progress. Re-evaluate yourself against the items in this list after six to eight months and record your progress. Keep working on achieving excellence in teaching in your college.

FOR WHOM IS THIS BOOK WRITTEN?

This book is written for three groups of academics/teachers.

- It is a self-help guide for medical and health professional teachers; that is the main intention.

- It is intended to help trainers, clinical course co-ordinators, directors of clinical skills laboratories and clinical deans to understand key principles of clinical teaching, monitor teachers, provide them with constructive feedback, and help them grow.

- It is an essential resource for directors of medical/health professional education departments, those involved in curriculum change and leading staff development and training programmes. The book can be an ideal resource in their work and help them to improve their training programmes.

References

1. Hansen PA, Roberts KB. Putting teaching back at the center. *Teaching and Learning in Medicine* 1992; **4**: 136–9.

2. Societal Needs Working Group, CanMEDS2000 Projects. Skills for the new millennium. *Annals of the Royal College of Physicians and Surgeons of Canada* 1996; **29**: 206–16.

3. Edgerton R, Hutchings P, Quinlan K. *The teaching portfolio: capturing the scholarship in teaching.* Washington, DC: American Association for Higher Education, 1991.

4. Mennin SP, McGrew MC. Scholarship in teaching and best evidence medical education synergy for teaching and learning. *Medical Teacher* 2000; **22**: 468–71.

5. Frank JR, Danoff D. The CanMEDS initiative: implementing an outcomes-based framework of physician competencies. *Medical Teacher* 2007; **29**: 642–7.

6. Snell L, Tallen S, Haist S *et al.* A review of the evaluation of clinical teaching: new perspectives and challenges. *Medical Education* 2000; **34**: 862–70.

7. Fincher R-ME, Simpson DE, Mennin SP *et al.* Scholarship in teaching: an imperative for the 21st century. *Academic Medicine* 2000; **75**: 887–94.

8. Hutchings P, Shulman LS. The scholarship of teaching new elaborations and developments. *Change* 1999; **31**: 11–15.

9. Boyer El. *Scholarship reconsidered: priorities of the professoriate.* Princeton, NJ: Carnegie Foundation for the Advancement of Teaching, 1990.

10. Moses AS, Heestand DE, Doyle LL, O'Sullivan PS. Impact of a teaching scholars program. *Academic Medicine* 2006; **81**: S89–S90.

11. Beckman TJ, Cook DA. Developing scholarly projects in education: a primer for medical teachers. *Medical Teacher* 2007; **20**: 210–18.

12. Goldszmidt MA, Zibrowski EM, Weston WW. Educational scholarship: it's not just a question of degree. *Medical Teacher* 2008; **30**: 34–9.

13. Glassick CE, Huber MR, Maeroff GI. *Scholarship assessed – evaluation of the professoriate.* San Francisco, CA: Jossey-Bass, 1997.

14. Glassick CE. Boyer's expanded definitions of scholarship, the standards of assessing scholarship and the elusiveness of the scholarship of teaching. *Academic Medicine* 2000; **75**: 877–80.

15. Simpson D, Fincher R-ME. Making a case for the teaching scholar. *Academic Medicine* 1999; **74**: 1296–9.

16. Lawrence DJ. A teaching scholar program in chiropractic education. *Journal of the Canadian Chiropractic Association* 2010; **54**: 17–23.

17. Medina M, Hammer D, Rose R *et al.* Demonstrating excellence in pharmacy teaching through scholarship. *Currents in Pharmacy Teaching and Learning* 2011; **3**: 255–9.

18. Klingensmith ME, Anderson KD. Educational scholarship as a route to academic promotion: a depiction of surgical education scholars. *American Journal of Surgery* 2006; **191**: 533–7.

19. Mennin SP. Standards for teaching in medical schools: double or nothing. *Medical Teacher* 1999; **21**: 543–5.

20. Van Der Vleuten C. Evidence-based education. *Advances in Physiology Education* 1995; **14**: S3.

21. Benor DE. Faculty development, teacher training and teacher accreditation in medical education: 20 years from now. *Medical Teacher* 2000; **33**: 503–12.

22. Mallon WT, Jones RF. How do medical schools use measurement systems to track faculty activity and productivity in teaching? *Academic Medicine* 2002; **77**: 115–23.

23. McGaghie WC. Scholarship, publication, and career advancement in health professions education: AMEE Guide No 43. *Medical Teacher* 2009; **31**: 574–90.

Further reading

Azer SA. The qualities of a good teacher: how can they be acquired and sustained? *Journal of the Royal Society of Medicine* 2005; **98**: 67–9.

Bligh J, Brice J. Further insights into the roles of the medical educator: the importance of scholarly management. *Academic Medicine* 2009; **84**: 1161–5.

Glassick CE. Reconsidering scholarship. *Journal of Public Health Management and Practise* 2000; **6**: 4–9.

Hart I. Best evidence medical education (BEME). *Medical Teacher* 1999; **21**: 453–4.

Hutchinson L. Evaluating and researching the effectiveness of educational interventions. *British Medical Journal* 1999; **318**: 1267–9.

Irby DM, Cooke M, Lowenstein D, Richards B. The academy movement: a structural approach to reinvigorating the education mission. *Academic Medicine* 2004; **79**: 729–36.

Jacelon CS, Donoghue LC, Breslin E. Scholar in residence: an innovative application of the scholarship of engagement. *Journal of Professional Nursing* 2010; **26**: 61–6.

Johnson-Farmer B, Frenn M. Teaching excellence: what great teachers teach us. *Journal of Professional Nursing* 2009; **25**: 267–72.

Marks ES. Defining scholarship at the uniformed services university of the health sciences school of medicine: a study in cultures. *Academic Medicine* 2000; **75**: 935–9.

Simpson D, Fincher R-ME, Hafler JP *et al.* Advancing educators and education by defining the components and evidence associated with educational scholarship. *Medical Educator* 2007; **41**: 1002–9.

CHAPTER 1

Be committed to your work

Teacher characteristics or attributes which are important to the learner include accessibility, enthusiasm, clarity, knowledge of discipline, role modelling, demonstrating clinical skills and taking the time for teaching.

DM Irby, 1987

1.1 Focus on the learning needs of your students
1.2 Work with passion
1.3 Uphold professional values
1.4 Be enthusiastic about clinical teaching and learning

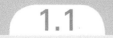

Focus on the learning needs of your students

Samy A Azer

Dr Lilly Ende joined the Department of General Practise a few months ago and has been asked to share in the teaching of third-year medical students. The Faculty of Medicine where she works introduced an integrated medical curriculum about three years ago and Early Clinical Exposure (ECE) has been established in the curriculum as a longitudinal module.

Dr Ende has no prior experience in integrated curricula. Instead of consulting with the co-ordinator of the ECE module, she designed her teaching session the same way she used to teach in a traditional medical curriculum. Because students were introduced to elements of clinical examination in years 1 and 2, her sessions were not building on what they already knew. Students were frustrated by her teaching sessions and felt that they were repeating what they already knew in this area.

CASE STUDY

This case raises an important issue about the need for teachers to address the needs of their students. Teachers may not explore this area prior to the preparation of their teaching session, and just focus on the contents they are interested in covering, from their point of view as the teacher. Such an approach will usually result in teaching sessions that do not meet the needs of the students and build on skills and knowledge they have already acquired.

Why is it important to know the learning needs of your students?

By identifying the learning needs of the students, teachers will be able to:

- Identify the knowledge and skills students have acquired already
- Understand the knowledge and skills students need to develop
- Establish the need and demand for their teaching/learning sessions
- Engage students in learning activities/tasks that allow them to add to the skills they have already developed
- Link teaching to practise
- Determine what design they will use in their teaching/learning sessions.

ACTION PLAN

To assess the student's learning needs, teachers need to:

- Become aware of the structure and design of the curriculum used and the modes of teaching/learning used
- Collect information about students' strengths and areas of need: look at evaluation reports, performance in assessment, as well as discuss with other teachers and the course co-ordinators the design and objectives of the course
- Use information collected to modify your learning/teaching sessions
- Plan strategies to implement in your sessions
- Don't introduce significant changes. Plan and gradually implement changes
- Ask students and colleagues to give you feedback on your teaching sessions

---

Take-home message

- Teachers have to design their teaching/learning sessions in a way that meets their students' learning needs.
- Understanding areas of strength and the needs/demands of your students is vital for optimum teaching and linking teaching to practise.

Further reading

Chan LK, Ip MS, Patil NG, Prosser M. Learning needs in a medical curriculum in Hong Kong. *Hong Kong Medical Journal* 2011; **17**: 202–7.

Haghparast N, Okubo M, Enciso R *et al*. Comparing student-generated learning needs with faculty objectives in PBL cases in dental education. *Journal of Dental Education* 2011; **75**: 1092–7.

Hesselgreaves H, Watson A, Crawford A *et al*. Medication safety: using incident date analysis and clinical focus groups to inform educational needs. *Journal of Evaluation in Clinical Practise* 2011 Nov doi:1111/j1365-2753 2011.01763x [Epub ahead of print].

Jest AD, Tonge A. Using a learning needs assessment to identify knowledge deficits regarding procedural sedation for paediatric patients. *AORN Journal* 2011; **94**: 567–74.

Work with passion

E Angela Chan

CASE SCENARIO: INSPIRING STUDENTS ABOUT THEIR PROFESSION

'I have witnessed how Ms Chan cares for the patient as a whole person and not only as a disease entity,' said Pamela. 'Working with a stroke patient, she helped us to learn about the reality that while some patients regain full function, many others do not. She showed us that helping people to improve their functioning and gain some independence is such a rewarding aspect of nursing. She is a great role model, but she expects us to be fully prepared for questions about our patient care. While she has high expectations, she provides us with her time and countless opportunities to learn with support. She believes in the potential in each of us to learn. I also recall a time when, faced with much opposition from other faculty members about our request for a fast-track summer programme, Ms Chan advocated for the students and volunteered her time to endeavour to meet our needs.'

CASE STUDY

Students love Ms Chan's enthusiasm and the sense of purpose that she has found in teaching. In her teaching, she enabled students to see the patient as a whole, and through her emphasis on making the best out of a situation, she instils optimism in her students to sustain their passion. Her approach of listening to and acknowledging students' needs without any collegial support again teaches students to pursue what may seem impossible in the face of adversity. Her high expectations of her students' performance, while being committed to helping them to succeed through recognition of their potential, has become imperative with regard to their motivation.

Why is it important to work with passion?

Students learn from their teachers, who work with passion, not only the knowledge and skills needed in caring for patients, but importantly an attitude – a love for nursing. For all teachers, the desired students' learning outcome is whether learning and understanding have been achieved as an attitude. Passion is one of the attitudes and attributes of competent teachers. Having passion in one's work transmits energy for others to believe, rendering the seemingly impossible possible, especially in the context of fiscal austerity. Our new generation of health professionals needs to be nurtured in their pursuit of passionate scholarship, in turn attracting and retaining the best to help negotiate the challenges.

What are the characteristics of working with passion?

Working with passion often translates into motivating students' continuous pursuit of their goals, nurturing inquisitive minds, and fostering self-directed learning. Passionate teachers set high standards for their students, matching these high expectations with support to reach those goals. The power of being a role model worthy of emulation comes from this commitment to teaching and, most of all, to the learner. From educational passion comes the sustained enthusiasm that is characteristic of effective teaching. Passionate teachers also live on the margins between what is known and not known, in turn allowing students to try new ideas and be creative.

ACTION PLAN

To work with passion in your group, consider the following actions.

- Appreciate students' efforts and believe in their potential. Being recognized and having the support to learn will motivate students in their continuous pursuit of the joys of learning and in facing the inherent challenges.

- Help students to think positively and be excited about learning new things, encourage new ideas and courageous leaps forward.

Take-home message

Working with passion helps to energize and motivate students' learning, providing a platform for grooming a future generation of competent and passionate professionals. Having developed certain core values of the meaning of being health professionals, they serve as a guide, helping students to navigate through often tumultuous health-care terrain.

Further reading

Hatem CJ, Searle NS, Gunderman R *et al.* The educational attributes and responsibilities of effective medical educators. *Academic Medicine* 2011; **86**: 474–80.

Wassermann S. *How I taught myself how to teach.* Boston, MA: Harvard Business School, 1983, case 3-383-016.

Uphold professional values

Gudrun Edgren and Margareta Troein

CASE SCENARIO: AFTER A SECOND OF THOUGHT

Dr Svensson and Thomas, a medical student, have spent the evening at the Accident and Emergency Department taking care of a never-ending line of patients. There have been few occasions for rest and just after midnight they enter a room where Mr Lundberg, aged 78, and his daughters are waiting. The daughters explain that their father has had a bad cough and become increasingly tired during the day. They also mention that he has diabetes (poorly controlled), hypertension and prostate hypertrophy. He has been a widower for four months and is depressed. Thomas takes a medical history and performs an examination, supplemented by Dr Svensson. She concludes that the patient suffers from pneumonia and his condition requires antibiotic treatment. The hospital is full and any overuse of beds has to go to patients with severe diseases. She offers a prescription and a return visit in a few days.

The daughters want their father to be admitted for treatment and observation. Dr Svensson patiently explains that he can be treated at home and that only patients with complicated conditions can be admitted, as there is a shortage of beds.

The daughters ask what kind of conditions Dr Svensson refers to, and she mentions diabetes and lung disease. Saying this, she realizes that Mr Lundberg has a typical complicating condition. After some consideration, she says to the patient and his daughters that she has made a mistake, apologizes and explains that her error is due to the hectic evening she has experienced at the hospital. Mr Lundberg is offered a hospital bed.

When Dr Svensson is alone with Thomas, they discuss what occurred.

CASE STUDY

Dr Svensson was about to make a mistake, thinking only about the pneumonia and forgetting about the patient's complicating condition, the diabetes. When confronted by the daughters she realized her mistake, which is obvious to the patient and his relatives. She risks losing face, which may mean embarrassment in the short run. However, she gains much more by upholding her professional values. The patient will be under good care if complications appear, the daughters accept that the doctor admitted her mistake, and the student has the opportunity to see a good role model with regard to handling mistakes he himself may make in the future.

The Medical Professionalism Project addressed the fundamental principles of medical professionalism which can be summarized under three main headings:

- Primacy of patient's welfare
- Patient's autonomy
- Social justice.

If Dr Svensson had not admitted her mistake, she would have violated these principles. Dr Svensson was working with a student and she had the added responsibility of acting as a good role model for the student. Role modelling is important for a student's learning of professional values, although professionalism must also be formally taught.

The professional responsibilities of the medical profession are a commitment to:

- Professional competence
- Honesty with patients
- Patient confidentiality
- Maintaining appropriate relationships with patients
- Improving quality of care
- Improving access to care
- Just distribution of finite resources
- Scientific knowledge
- Maintaining trust by managing conflicts of interest
- Professional responsibilities.

ACTION PLAN

As a clinical teacher you must, like all doctors, uphold professional values, as well as teach your students to do so. Also you can do this by:

- Being aware of and respecting professional values
- Being prepared to admit your mistakes
- Realizing that you are always a role model for your students
- Stimulating reflection, both for yourself and your students
- Arranging formal teaching, e.g. group discussions.

> ### Take-home message
>
> - Uphold professional values. Remember, you are always a role model as a professional for your students.
> - Admit your mistakes if you make any.

Further reading

ABIM Foundation. American Board of Internal Medicine; ACP-ASIM Foundation. American College of Physicians–American Society of Internal Medicine; European Federation of Internal Medicine. Medical professionalism in the new millennium: a physician charter. *Annals of Internal Medicine* 2002; **136**: 243–6.

Cohen JJ, Cruess S, Davidson C. Alliance between society and medicine. The public's stake in medical professionalism. *Journal of the American Medical Association* 2007; **298**: 670–3.

Cruess SR, Cruess RL, Steinert Y. Role modelling – making the most of a powerful teaching strategy. *British Medical Journal* 2008; **336**: 718–21.

Medical Professionalism Project. Medical professionalism in the new millennium: a physicians' charter. *Lancet* 2002; **395**: 520–2.

Passi V, Doug M, Peile E *et al.* Developing medical professionalism in future doctors: a systematic review. *International Journal of Medical Education* 2010; **1**: 19–29.

Be enthusiastic about clinical teaching and learning

Sam Leinster

Sam Leinster

CASE SCENARIO: IMPRESSED BY HIS INTERACTIVE RELATIONSHIP

Dr Bell, a physician in the teaching hospital, is recognized by all his colleagues as a highly competent and knowledgeable clinician. He constantly receives excellent evaluations from the students for his teaching. He has been nominated on several occasions for teaching awards. You sit in on one of his clinical teaching sessions and are impressed by his interactive relationship with the students and by his evident interest in the patients and their conditions. The students tell you that they enjoy his teaching sessions because he makes medicine seem exciting.

CASE STUDY

The reason that the students appreciate Dr Bell's teaching so much is almost certainly his enthusiasm.

Studies of the characteristics that make a good teacher regularly identify enthusiasm as important. Techniques for appearing enthusiastic in a classroom setting can be learnt and draw on lessons from the acting profession. Transmitting enthusiasm in the clinical setting requires a rather different approach.

Sutkin *et al.* in a review of studies of the characteristics of a good clinical teacher found that enthusiastic teachers displayed three components of enthusiasm – enthusiasm for medicine, enthusiasm for teaching and being an enthusiastic person in general.

Enthusiasm for medicine

In order to be effective, the teacher needs to have a thorough knowledge of the subject matter that they are dealing with. In the clinical setting, this means keeping up to date with the latest developments in the field. Without this, clinical practise will become routine and repetitive, the care of patients will suffer and teaching will become dull and boring. The teacher who is constantly seeking to increase their knowledge invites the students to join him or her in the adventure of learning. The students gradually come to see that medicine is not a finite body of knowledge that they will one day be able to master, but an unending quest that can provide intellectual stimulation for the rest of their lives.

Enthusiasm for teaching

A major part of the enjoyment of teaching comes from the interaction with the students and the willingness to receive from the students, as well as to give to them. If you regard teaching as one-way traffic where you, the teacher, deliver wisdom and knowledge to an entirely passive group of students you will rapidly burn out. If you get to know them as individuals and engage in dialogue with them you will enter a relationship that will generate enthusiasm in you and in the students. It is unlikely that you will remain enthusiastic for teaching unless you actively engage with the students. Enthusiasm for teaching can also be conveyed in simple things like never missing a teaching session and always being punctual.

Being an enthusiastic person

Maintaining enthusiasm for teaching is easier if your approach to life in general is enthusiastic. The most dedicated teachers are very often those with a wide range of interests beyond their professional duties.

ACTION PLAN

Enthusiasm can be developed and sustained by:

- Keeping up to date with your clinical discipline
- Engaging actively with the students, recognizing that you can learn from them, as well as teach them
- Exploring fresh approaches to teaching in discussion with senior and junior colleagues
- Maintaining a wide range of interests outside medicine.

Take-home message

Enthusiastic teachers are effective teachers.

Further reading

Metcalfe A, Game A. The teacher's enthusiasm. *Australian Educational Researcher* 2006; **33**: 91–106.

Sutkin G, Wagner E, Harris I, Schiffer R. What makes a good clinical teacher in medicine? A review of the literature. *Academic Medicine* 2008; **83**: 452–66.

CHAPTER 2

Encourage an open and trusting environment

The good teacher creates a positive learning environment.
L Snell *et al.*, 2000

Create a climate of trust

Samy A Azer

CASE SCENARIO: LOOKING FOR A NEW WAY

'I've had enough of these comments,' said Monika, storming out of the classroom. Monika and several other students in the class felt that Mrs Robinson, their teacher, had a terrible habit of viciously attacking students and highlighting their mistakes in a degrading manner. She always claims that it is part of her teaching responsibilities to provide feedback to students about their performance. Once she said to one of her colleagues, 'Students will always learn better and will remember their teacher's feedback if they are embarrassed'. Last week, she repeatedly asked her students about a folder she lost and insinuated that one of them may have, accidentally, taken it. It turned out a few days later that she had misplaced it in her room.

Students hate her classes and find it difficult to work with her. Recently, Mrs Robinson reported that several students were absent from class and some of them had not shown up for the last few days.

CASE STUDY

In this case, the teacher needlessly insulted and alienated students in her class. The teacher's pattern of criticizing her students caused Monika and others to avoid her classes. When necessary, it is important for a teacher to give feedback. However, the way teachers provide feedback is of the utmost importance. You need to think about delivering feedback in a way that builds up members in the group and provides opportunities for teachers to strengthen their relationship with their students. Asking students questions in a way that shows doubt or a lack of trust could have disastrous outcomes and diminish the rapport you have built with them.

Why is it important to create a climate of trust?

Creation of a climate of trust will free your students from fears and will encourage them to express their own thoughts and ideas even if they are not correct or unsure about their answers. A climate of trust will enhance students' engagement and contribution to the class discussion and will allow them to enjoy what they are doing.

What are the characteristics of a climate of trust in a classroom?

- Teachers treat individual students as assets to their class, and their attitudes are consistent and not conditioned by students' behaviour.
- Teachers are able to attract students to their classes and to the subject they teach.
- The climate of learning shows mutual respect, interest and a willingness to work.
- In such an environment, no one feels blamed, hurt or accused, and the general feeling in the classroom is that everyone is treated equally and fairly.

ACTION PLAN

To create a climate of trust in your group, consider the following actions.

- Encouragement always fosters a safe environment. On the other hand, teachers who belittle students run the risk of losing those students, not only as part of their team but also as motivated long-term learners.
- It is always useful to think before giving feedback to students, especially when giving negative feedback. Consider the impact that may occur because of your comments and whether your comments will benefit or possibly cause harm.
- If you have negative feedback for a student, save it for a private session.
- Always think about the best strategies to deliver feedback and how to 'put your words' in a win-win approach. Always deliver your comments/feedback in the right place and at the right time.

Take-home message

- Your ability to trust others working with you grows with your own motives to trust yourself.
- One of the basic missions of a teacher is to build trust in their relationships with their students. Without trust, their effort will be wasted and they will never achieve their potential in fostering the learner's needs.

Further reading

Brookfield SD. *The skillful teacher: on technique, trust and responsiveness in the classroom.* San Francisco, CA: Jossey-Bass, 2000.

Shaw RB. *Trust in the balance: building successful organizations on results, integrity and concern.* San Francisco, CA: Jossey-Bass, 1997.

Encourage your students to learn from their mistakes

Samy A Azer

CASE SCENARIO: PUSHING THE GROUP DISCUSSION

For the last three weeks, the teacher has noticed that his small group is slow in the discussion of their clinical cases. Students were not able to complete the discussion of the whole case and left parts incomplete.

The teacher felt unhappy with his group's approach and thought he could discuss this issue with them. He arrived late and was unable to stop the discussion. He thought he could discuss his concern with them at the end of the tutorial. Because of the tediousness of their discussion, he decided to push them and interpret their discussion so that they could complete the case discussion in the allocated time.

Things went wrong and his students did not understand why their teacher was interfering a great deal and interrupting their discussion. They felt that there was a struggle between them, and the tutorials became unproductive. Two students left the tutorial early. The teacher felt that his students were a little bit angry at his constant interruption of their discussion and thus decided to postpone his discussion with them.

CASE STUDY

In this case, the teacher did not discuss his concerns immediately. Even when he decided to discuss his concerns, with his class, he was late and unprepared. Changing his approach by interfering and pushing the discussion was not appreciated by his students and caused more confusion in the group. It appears that he had no plan in his approach and continued to delay the discussion of this problem with his group. The teacher should have used the last 10–15 minutes to discuss issues like this. The teacher should consult with the group and encourage them to own the problem and strategize on the actions they should undertake to find a solution.

Why is it important to train students to learn from their mistakes?

People, when supported, look at things differently when they make mistakes. They may think about creative solutions. Therefore, it is important that learners be encouraged to face their mistakes, and be trained on how to work on improving their performance in areas of weakness. When students work on their mistakes and gradually master these areas, they will become more confident, and their perception of failure will change as a result.

What strategies will you use to achieve your goals?

- Tell students that we are all learning and it is acceptable to make mistakes.
- Create an environment that perceives mistakes to be an opportunity for learning.
- Keep thinking about innovative ways that allow students to see their mistakes as an opportunity to think about new options.
- Develop the habit of giving and receiving feedback with your students.

ACTION PLAN

To ensure that your students learn from their mistakes, consider the following actions.

- Bring their mistakes to their attention and encourage them to identify these shortcomings. Open-ended questions that could foster such a discussion may include: (1) How do you think you are doing? (2) What are the things you are doing well? (3) What are the things you need to achieve/improve? (4) How important is this to you? (5) What strategies do we need to take to achieve these goals? and (6) What do you think you could do until we meet again?
- Avoid throwing the problems/mistakes onto your students. Support and facilitate the discussion so that they can realize that there is a problem and can use a strategic plan to improve their performance.
- Ask your students to continue to monitor their action plan and consider whether they are able to implement their plan and achieve their goals or not and effectively identify what changes they could make to their plan, if need be.

> ## Take-home message
>
> - To help students learn from their mistakes, you need to tell them that it is acceptable to make mistakes.
> - Help to create an environment that sees mistakes as a way of learning.

Further reading

Dillon C. *Learning from mistakes in clinical practise.* Pacific Grove, CA: Brooks/Cole, 2003.

Finn JA. *Getting a PhD. Routledge study guide.* New York: Routledge Taylor & Francis Group, 2005.

Help students redefine failure as a learning experience

Onishi Hirotaka

CASE SCENARIO

Miki, a fifth-year medical student, came to the family medicine department and had her first independent consultation with a real outpatient, a 35-year-old man complaining of chest pain. She started the consultation with greeting words and open-ended questions as she had practised in the 'Introduction to clinical medicine' curriculum, but noticed that she did not understand what kind of closed questions she should ask. She skipped the closed questions and continued the medical interview with past history, family history, social history and closing. She asked the patient to stay in the waiting room until a preceptor would call him again to the consultation room. After her presentation of the case, the preceptor gave her feedback: 'Miki, you did not have comprehensive differential diagnoses to ask closed questions for this patient'. Miki felt ashamed of her lack of clinical knowledge.

CASE STUDY

This scenario describes the first attempt at independent outpatient consultation by a fifth-year medical student. Usually, such students have a certain amount of clinical knowledge, but a large part is not organized to be practically useful in a clinical setting.

Reflective practise for the next session

Miki needs to reflect on her first attempt at consultation from the point of view of clinical reasoning. Normally, clinical knowledge is taught and learned in the direction from a diagnosis to its related signs/symptoms, but clinical reasoning is conducted from signs/symptoms to a diagnosis. Reorganization of information in the brain will be needed for a successful medical interview to achieve better clinical reasoning.

How to teach in an outpatient department and provide feedback on a failure experience

The preceptor provided comments for feedback. Confrontation is effective to allow a learner to appreciate what she/he did not notice but in this case, she is already aware that she did not know what to ask in closed questions. Some learners might be embarrassed by the confrontation comments. Instead, the preceptor should ask how she intended to ask questions and how she would change the medical interview for the next time. Furthermore, the preceptor should consider if a student is ready for outpatient consultation. Insecurities may intimidate learners and lead to systematic failure, which may lead to deterioration of the learning process.

Significant event analysis

'Significant event analysis (SEA)' is a useful technique used to develop constructive reflection with a group of students. SEA has the power to change such a significant event into an unforgettable learning experience through the group reflection process. SEA sometimes evokes emotions of, for example, anger and sadness. If team members successfully address the emotional conflict and the significant events of a presenter, the team will become more comfortable with future learning.

SEA processes include: (1) description of the significant event; (2) initial thoughts and emotions; (3) what was done well; (4) what requires improvement; (5) what should have been done; and (6) action plans for the future. The most important point of SEA for the preceptor is to ensure that a *blame culture* is not created. If the preceptor blames or critically assesses the presenter, he/she might become uncomfortable and the audience will be negatively affected as well.

ACTION PLAN

To help students redefine failure as a learning experience:

- Facilitate the learner to reflect on what was done well and what needs improvement. Students can usually change a failure into a learning experience
- Significant event analysis is a systematic method for reflection by a team of learners.

> Take-home message
>
> - Failure or error is a valuable opportunity for reflective learning. Good teachers can change a failure into a positive learning experience.

Further reading

Davies HTO, Nutley SM. Developing learning organisations in the new NHS. *British Medical Journal* 2000; **320**: 998–1001.

Henderson E, Berlin A, Freeman G, Fuller J. Twelve tips for promoting significant event analysis to enhance reflection in undergraduate medical students. *Medical Teacher* 2002; **24**: 121–4.

Accept uncertainty in medicine

Subha Ramani

CASE SCENARIO: THE UNDIAGNOSED CHEST PAIN

A 45-year-old patient was admitted to hospital with severe chest pain for three days. The ward team consists of a consultant, two residents and two medical students. Student John admitted the patient with resident Chris. Based on differential diagnoses of angina, oesophageal reflux and costochondritis, work-up included a chest x-ray, electrocardiograph (ECG) and blood tests. On rounds, John informed the patient that all investigations were normal and there was no evidence of a heart attack or anything serious. The patient asked, 'If it is not a heart attack, what is it?' John was stumped and looked at Chris. Chris reiterated that it was not a heart attack, but did not provide the answer the patient was looking for. The patient asked, 'Why are you discharging me without an answer?'

CASE STUDY

In this case, the medical team forms a diagnostic hypothesis based on patient presentation and conducts investigations accordingly. Their differential diagnoses have been excluded by history, examination and investigations. They are faced with diagnostic uncertainty, and their subsequent explanations to the patient are considered unsatisfactory. Although this case highlights trainees' encounters with medical uncertainty, many senior clinicians find it equally difficult to acknowledge uncertainty and verbalize the words 'I do not know' to trainees or patients.

Why is it important to accept uncertainty in medicine?

Uncertainty may be reduced by up-to-date knowledge, but cannot be eliminated from clinical decision making. Thus, intuition guides decisions resulting in biases and heuristics that can distort the decision-making process. Physicians and students are frequently unaware of uncertainty and resulting biases. Non-acceptance of uncertainty can result in multiple tests being ordered and marked variability in treatment. Educating students about uncertainty and resulting biases is crucial. Teachers must serve as role models during patient interactions, debrief and discuss strategies to deal with uncertainty.

What are the sources of medical uncertainty?

- Technical sources of uncertainty arise when there is insufficient information to predict effects of interventions or prognosis, e.g. knowledge not up to date, variability in biological processes.
- Personal sources of uncertainty occur within the doctor–patient relationship when the patient's wishes are unclear or cannot be incorporated.
- Conceptual sources of uncertainty arise from limited resources, general guidelines being adapted for individual patients or past experiences guiding management.

What are the responses to medical uncertainty?

- Unawareness or denial of uncertainty.
- Doing what their colleagues do – medical orthodoxy.
- Not disclosing uncertainties to patients to avoid losing dominance in decision making.
- Increased action – ordering more tests, more admissions.
- Intolerance for uncertainty transmitted to students, leading them to prefer high technology specialties and negativity towards geriatric, psychiatric or chronic pain patients.
- Using vague descriptions of likelihood such as 'probably' and 'possibly' to patients, subject to varied interpretations by doctors and patients.

ACTION PLAN

To prepare young doctors, teachers should create a climate facilitating awareness of uncertainty.

- Educating students about uncertainty in medicine and biases in clinical decision making to provide insights into diagnoses and management.
- Teaching students evidence-based medicine to reduce technical uncertainty.
- Admit limitations in knowledge, acknowledge uncertainty in management decisions to both students and patients.

Take-home message

- Uncertainty is inevitable in clinical decisions, leading to intuition playing a prominent role in patient management.
- Physicians might react to uncertainty by unawareness or denial, leading to errors and biases in decision making.
- A thorough history and clinical examination rather than more investigations usually helps in dealing with uncertainty.
- Medical curricula should include evidence-based medicine, educating students about medical uncertainty, clinical reasoning strategies, disclosure of uncertainty to patients and the importance of shared clinical decision making.

Further reading

Azer SA. Commentary: Lessons on functional diseases. *British Medical Journal* 2006; **333**: 135.

Ghosh AK. On the challenges of using evidence-based information: the role of clinical uncertainty. *Journal of Laboratory and Clinical Medicine* 2004; **144**: 60–4.

Ghosh AK. Understanding medical uncertainty: a primer for physicians. *Journal of the Association of Physicians of India* 2004; **52**: 739–42.

Hall HH. Reviewing intuitive decision-making and uncertainty: the implications for medical education. *Medical Education* 2002; **36**: 216–24.

Be accessible/available to students

Subha Ramani

CASE SCENARIO: A DYSFUNCTIONAL SMALL GROUP

A junior teacher was tutoring eight medical students in an eight-week clinical problem-solving course with weekly 120-minute sessions. Staff orientation for problem-based learning (PBL) tutors emphasized student autonomy and self-directed learning. The tutor allowed students to do all the talking. Two dominant students took over the sessions, listing learning goals, reading topics and learning assignments and three students were silent. The teacher felt that learning assignments did not cover all of the important topics and the group process was dysfunctional. The students felt that the teacher did not provide guidance in directing the clinical questions and learning assignments, and was unavailable after tutorials for questions and clarifications.

CASE STUDY

In this case, the teacher did not possess sufficient experience and/or was not trained adequately in small group facilitation. Although he allowed students to lead the sessions, he did not know when to interrupt and redirect, prevent the dominant students from taking over and engage all learners. He was seen as not approachable since students did not perceive his skills of listening, questioning or responding to questions. He was seen as unavailable as he did not encourage students to contact him after hours.

Why are teacher accessibility and availability important?

Recent changes in medical education emphasize self-directed learning with students taking responsibility for their learning. Assessment methods have moved to performance-based and multisource assessment. The move from a teacher-centred to a student-centred learning environment focuses on students' learning goals and plans rather than the teacher's style or content delivery. A good teacher today is one who facilitates student learning.

Definition of accessibility and availability

Medical educators cannot spend large amounts of time with their students. In clinical settings, they often meet briefly after patient encounters to discuss specific aspects of cases. However, the quantity of time with students is not as important as its quality. The definitions below show accessibility and availability as distinct entities.

Availability refers to a teacher who is willing to stay back after the session, answers paged messages and emails promptly and courteously and allows adequate time for teaching.

Accessibility may be a more global entity aimed at the establishment of a non-threatening learning environment including effective communication and a perception that a teacher is approachable, encourages questions for clarification, facilitates desired student interaction and relates to students by being sensitive to their needs.

How do accessibility and availability relate to the learning environment?

In studies exploring medical trainees' opinions on excellent teachers, knowledge and cognitive skills took second place to non-cognitive skills, such as enthusiasm, communication skills and other personality traits, skills that promote a favourable learning atmosphere.

Specific skills include:

- Establishing rapport
- Making eye contact
- Speaking clearly
- Being available outside set class times
- Encouraging clarifying questions
- Helping students develop learning goals
- Excellent listening and speaking skills
- Encouraging active participation

- Answering questions carefully and precisely
- Questioning students in a non-threatening manner.

ACTION PLAN

- Elicit students' learning goals and plans, ensure their appropriateness to achieve learning outcomes.
- Coach and facilitate learning and do not provide all the information and answers.
- Be available after hours to answer questions and guide learning goals and plans.

Take-home message

- Medical education today emphasizes student autonomy and self-directed learning.
- Teachers need to be facilitators of student learning rather than repositories of information.
- Students need guidance from teachers as they define learning goals and make learning plans.
- For effective self-directed learning, teachers must be available to answer questions, provide resources and ensure that learning goals and plans are appropriate.
- Accessibility includes skills such as listening, speaking clearly, actively engaging all students and non-threatening questioning.
- Staff development is crucial in helping teachers develop these skills.

Further reading

Buchel TM, Edwards FD. Characteristics of effective clinical teachers. *Family Medicine* 2005; **37**: 30–5.

Dent J, Harden RM. *A practical guide for medical teachers*, 3rd edn. London: Churchill Livingstone, 2009.

Harden RM, Crosby J. AMEE Guide No 20: The good teacher is more than a lecturer: the twelve roles of the teacher. *Medical Teacher* 2000; **22**: 334–47.

McLean M. Qualities attributed to an ideal educator by medical students: should faculty take cognizance? *Medical Teacher* 2001; **23**: 367–70.

Sutkin G, Wagner E, Harris I, Schiffer R. What makes a good clinical teacher in medicine? A review of the literature. *Academic Medicine* 2008; **83**: 452–66.

CHAPTER 3

Interact and communicate with respect

Students expect and deserve to find warm and enthusiastic faculty who will teach, guide (communicate) and support them on their journey.

B Johnson-Farmer and M Frenn, 2009

3.1 Communicate effectively with others
3.2 Encourage input from others and give credit for contribution
3.3 Act with integrity
3.4 Provide a model for professional ethical standards
3.5 Show a caring attitude

Communicate effectively with others

Samy A Azer

CASE SCENARIO: SHOULD WE TALK ABOUT OUR CONCERNS?

Rachel, a science student, was talking with Sarah, another student in her group. 'Sarah, did you notice what happened with our teacher today?' said Rachel. 'It was unbelievable!' Sarah exclaimed. 'I was just thinking about it. Did you notice how many times he ignored the points raised by Lydia, Victoria and Glen?'

'It was so disappointing. He also repeated what we had already discussed. I can't see the point of his questions. I am not sure if he really listens to our group discussion and follows up what we say,' Rachel added.

'Sometimes he seems a little absent minded and thoughtful. I do not think he realizes the damage he causes when he just tries to enforce some information and ignores our discussion points,' Sarah agreed.

'Do you think we should talk to him about our concerns?' asked Rachel. Sarah simply shrugged.

CASE STUDY

One of the critical components of the communication process is listening effectively. This case scenario raises a number of communication problems:

- Ignoring points raised by students
- Failing to follow up on what was said by group members
- Interrupting the discussion for no obvious reason
- Poor timing of interruption
- Focusing on what you want to say and ignoring students' input
- Causing frustration and possibly confusion due to poor communication.

Why is it important to communicate effectively with others?

- To ensure optimal outcomes
- To avoid/minimize conflict
- To establish great relationships
- To minimize errors and ensure safety
- To invest in time and minimize time wasting
- To achieve your goals in a win-win approach

What are the barriers to effective communication?

- The choice of words, which influence the overall quality of the communication
- Misleading body language, tone of voice or the use of non-verbal forms of communication
- Relationships, past experience and cultural differences
- State of mind, situation and timing
- Interpersonal relationships
- Inconsistent statements, lack of evidence, lack of clarity and the use of jargon
- Over-interpretation of what is said
- Lack of listening
- Focusing on personal views and missing objectivity
- Focusing on the fine details and ignoring the big picture
- Assuming that others see the situation in the same way you do

What do effective communicators do?

- Look at the person, listen and respond in a way that shows understanding and interest
- Do not dominate the conversation
- React to the message appropriately
- Do not try to change the topic to something that interests them
- Be aware of the body language used and non-verbal clues

- Check for understanding and ask good questions that clarify issues and ensure understanding
- Use skills and strategies to ensure they comprehend issues discussed
- Appreciate what is said and show empathy
- Be descriptive, non-judgemental or threatening in their approach

ACTION PLAN

To have effective communication with your students, consider the following action plans:

- Concentrate on what the speaker is saying
- Focus on the issues raised and flow of the discussion
- Do not be distracted by the speaker's voice, accent, gender or ethnicity
- Clarify issues you do not understand but do not try to shift the discussion to your own interest and personal views
- Listening well to what is said usually ensures better communication.

Take-home message

- Everyone needs to improve the effectiveness of his or her communication skills.
- The key to effective communication is good listening.

Further reading

Chambers HE. *Effective communication skills for scientific and technical professionals*. Jackson, TN: Perseus Books Group, 2003.

Cooper PJ, Simonds CJ. *Communication for the classroom teacher*, 7th edn. Boston: Allyn & Bacon, 2003.

Nichols RG, Stevens LA, Bartolome F, Argyris C. *Harvard business review on effective communication*. Harvard: Harvard Business School Press, 1999.

Encourage input from others and give credit for contribution

Samy A Azer

CASE SCENARIO: WHEN NO CREDIT IS GIVEN

Stephanie Lambert is a recently trained teacher from the school of physiotherapy. She is teaching second-year students and today she is doing her fourth tutorial. During the first three tutorials, it appears that Stephanie has encouraged three students to dominate the group discussion. Despite being trained to become a small group facilitator in a student-centred curriculum, she appears to take on the role of a traditional teacher. She only accepts right answers. Students who provide wrong answers feel unwelcome when contributing further to the group discussion.

On several occasions, Stephanie does not acknowledge the contribution of members in her group. Even when students do a good job, she does not acknowledge the achievement made. She usually interferes, adding more factual knowledge. Those who give wrong answers are questioned by saying 'Really?', 'Who told you that?', 'That is not correct …', or 'I do not agree at all …'.

Her approach suppresses most students in her group and has created an unhealthy environment. Students want to end the tutorial and leave early.

CASE STUDY

The lack of acknowledgement of contribution and the failure to encourage students to contribute to the discussion could result in frustration and group malfunction. Frustration such as this is certain to occur particularly in classes where teachers use inappropriate teaching approaches. Failure of the teachers to give credit when students contribute could affect the group discussion, resulting in:

CASE STUDY (continued)

- Poor student contribution to the discussion
- Lack of interest in participating
- Creation of an unhealthy environment and a sense of lacking security
- Poor group communication
- Lacking interest in learning and poor engagement.

Why is giving credit to students for their contribution useful?

When praise is given when it has been earned:

- It enhances student's performance
- It fosters their engagement
- It enables them to achieve their potential
- It keeps them working with energy and purpose
- It builds a safe and a healthy environment
- It encourages co-operation.

ACTION PLAN

Teachers who open the discussion and encourage students to evaluate different options, search for new information, and weigh the evidence for and against each hypothesis are in fact encouraging their students to learn. Rewarding students' contribution whenever they think, interpret, evaluate, ask good questions and contribute to construction of information delivered by the group is vital. What is more important in this process is not just the pieces of factual knowledge they need to know, but rather students' effort in achieving these learning qualities.

To establish a rewarding culture with your students, consider the following action plans.

- Always say 'Thank you' or 'You've done an excellent job' when a student in your class contributes.
- Do not be excessive but be wise about the need to encourage your students in an appropriate manner.

- Accept the views of all students and never be the 'policeman' who judges their views. Instead, encourage them to think and evaluate different perspectives.

- Encourage a system with your students where you debate issues on the basis of evidence rather than being dependent on you for the answers.

> ## Take-home message
>
> - Use praise when it has been earned.
> - When you give praise to students, identify what was good about what was done, why it was good, and in what way their contribution positively impacted the group's work.

Further reading

Cooper PJ, Simonds CJ. *Communication for the classroom teacher*, 7th edn. Columbus, OH: Allyn & Bacon, 2003.

Holmes W. *The heart of a teacher: true stories of inspiration and encouragement*. Ada, MI: Bethany House Publishers, 2002.

Act with integrity

Samy A Azer

CASE SCENARIO: HE IS ALSO MY TEACHER

Dr David Morgan, a clinical teacher, has recently been invited to be a member of the Objective Structured Clinical Examination (OSCE) committee responsible for writing the examination questions for years 4 and 5. Dr Morgan has recently established a relationship with Lee, a fifth-year medical student and they plan to get married next year. Dr David asked Lee not to mention anything about their relationship as he feels that his position as a clinical teacher may cause some conflict of interest. Lee agreed to his request and kept their relationship as a secret, even her close friends didn't know about it. Dr Morgan sees Lee regularly outside the workplace. It is the night of her OSCE and Lee feels stressed. She calls Dr Morgan to help her as she prepares for the examination.

CASE STUDY

This case raises an important issue about maintaining a professional attitude and acting with integrity. Dr Morgan's behaviour is unethical and he should have declared to the OSCE committee that there was a conflict of interest, and thus, he should not be involved in writing examination questions at least for this year. Although it is not clear from the case scenario whether he has mentioned to his fiancée that he is a member of the OSCE committee, his agreement in helping Lee prepare for her examination is another source of conflict of interest and a breach of integrity as a teacher.

Why is it important for a teacher to act with integrity?

Integrity for a teacher may comprise a number of aspects.

- **Integrity in knowledge**. A teacher should show appreciation for the relative disposition of things, and their relationships, regardless of what he/she may wish to be the case.

- **Integrity in research**. A teacher should seek scholarly outcomes and be keen about exploring pieces of information that help humanity and future research, rather than pursuing his/her own personal views.

- **Integrity in teaching**. A teacher should aim at enhancing students' critical thinking skills and their professional attitude rather than providing them with pieces of information about his/her subject.

- **Integrity in building students up**. A teacher should demonstrate interest in building his/her students up, monitoring their progress, providing them with constructive feedback, and keeping them engaged to reach their potential.

- **Integrity in relationships**. A teacher should be keen to build healthy and professional relationships with his/her students, colleagues, patients and community.

- **Integrity in assessment**. A teacher should assess students using valid and reliable tools. He/she should enable students to learn from their mistakes and encourage them to reflect on their learning.

ACTION PLAN

- Practise the professional code of ethics in your day-to-day activities.

- Always strive to demonstrate integrity, morality and virtue in your interactions and relationships with your students, patients, colleagues and the wider community.

- If you are facing a grey area and are not sure what to do, ask a reliable senior colleague for advice.

Take-home message

- Clinical teachers are expected to be moral, ethical and demonstrate integrity and a professional attitude in their relationship with their students, patients, people working with them and the wider community.

- As professionals, teachers may not always meet all of the conditions required of them, but must continually strive to do so. Detraction from integrity, morality and virtue may lead to legal consequences and a loss of reputation and career.

Further reading

Dudzinski DM. Integrity in the relationship between medical ethics and professionalism. *American Journal of Bioethics* 2004; **4**: 26–7.

Hutchins B, Cobb S. When will we be ready for academic integrity? *Journal of Dental Education* 2008; **72**: 359–63.

Meehan E. A concept of professionalism; integrity and openness. *World of Irish Nursing* 1975; **4**: 4–5.

Miller FG, Brody H. Viewpoint: professional integrity in industry-sponsored clinical trials. *Academic Medicine* 2005; **80**: 899–904.

Sullivan W. *Work and integrity: the crisis and promise of professionalism in North America*. New York: Harper Collins, 1995.

Provide a model for professional ethical standards

Zubair Amin

CASE SCENARIO: AN OBLIGING ACADEMIC

You have joined a new medical school just few months ago as an assistant professor. As a young academic working for a prestigious institute, you are determined to uphold the highest ethical standard in teaching and clinical practise. As a part of the university's orientation to new teachers you were given a 'code of conduct' for the academic staff, which spells out, in broad terms, the role and responsibilities of a teacher.

Recently, your head of department approached you to serve as a question developer for the final-year Objective Structured Clinical Examination (OSCE). This is your first experience in OSCE. As a student you never had similar examinations. As an obliging academic trying not to offend the superior, you reluctantly agreed to take up the role. You developed an OSCE station which was implemented without much change in the final examination.

However, during the post-examination review of the station, you realize that some of the items in the OSCE checklist were interpreted differently by different examiners. This resulted in a great variability in marking. Several students failed in that OSCE station. Although the students passed the entire examination despite their failure in this particular OSCE, you feel you have a duty to respond. However, you are unsure how to go about doing this. In particular, you are concerned that revealing the mistake to the Assessment Committee might embarrass the head of the department who also shares the responsibility of maintaining quality in the examination.

CASE STUDY

The role of clinical teachers includes being a skilled assessor. In this role, a clinical teacher is expected to perform several inter-related tasks, such as planning an examination, developing/ writing a question, conducting an examination and serving as an examiner. Too often, such roles are delegated to the clinical teacher without appropriate training and briefing. This particular scenario, in many variations, is commonplace in academia. A typical code of conduct might give clinical teachers some general guidelines about the role and responsibilities, but might not be sufficiently detailed to deal with individual dilemmas as depicted in the scenario.

In your opinion, what are the professional ethical standards that a medical teacher should uphold?

In a complex environment like clinical medicine, a medical teacher has multiple roles, including being an information provider, role model, facilitator, teacher, assessor, resource developer and planner. In a given time, a medical teacher might take up one or several of these roles. The professional standards and ethical values governing the roles vary, depending on the roles and context of the work. Thus, it is useful to develop a set of guiding principles that act as an internal ethical compass for an individual that should include duties as an examiner, responsibility as a clinical teacher in conflicted situations, and professional obligation to remain well trained in the task provided.

How do you resolve the conflict of interest described above?

While there is no absolute right and wrong answer in dealing with ethical dilemmas, it is important to recognize the consequences of a given action and inaction. It is imperative that student centricity in education is not limited to concept and declaration only; it should be translated into practise. In this situation, the students were the ultimate sufferers even though this did not result in any major failures. This should be resolved with students in mind that might include recalibration of marks or removal of the faulty station. Second, the medical teacher and the head of the department should agree upon a joint action plan to prevent further recurrence of similar problems which must include proper faculty training and briefing before assigning a task to the subordinate. The responsibility of the head of department is to provide necessary support for the clinical teacher to attend such faculty development programmes. Conversely, it is the clinical teacher's professional and ethical responsibility to keep up to date with faculty development in the given area of work.

ACTION PLAN

- Review the institutional code of conduct for teachers; if a code of conduct is unavailable, lobby for developing one.
- Compare ethical guidelines and codes of conduct for teachers from various sources; include sources beyond medical schools and universities.
- Proactively train to become more efficient and skilled as a clinical teacher.

Take-home message

- Ethical dilemmas are commonplace in education; many are ignored or not pursued further.
- In ethical dilemmas, it is vitally important to define the core issue and identify the consequences to various stakeholders.
- In the presence of multiple stakeholders with conflicting viewpoints and agendas, it might be useful to identify the primary stakeholders affected.

Further reading

Harden RM, Crosby JR. The good teacher is more than a lecturer: the twelve roles of the teacher. *Medical Teacher* 2004; **22**: 334–47.

Show a caring attitude

Samy A Azer and Rana Hassanato

CASE SCENARIO: MY TEACHER CARES FOR US

In an alumni party, Dr Allan Moore was invited together with over 30 alumni who graduated 50 years ago. Dr Moore was a consultant and professor of gynaecology and obstetrics in the same university and a number of his students attended the celebration. During the celebration, a number of Dr Moore's students talked about his caring attitude and how he used to look after his students and provide excellent care to his patients and people working with him. They also talked about the impact of his caring attitude on them and how his care changed their lives.

CASE STUDY

This case highlights how teachers make an impact on their students and how their caring attitude changed their lives. A caring attitude cannot be taught in a lecture or through reading a textbook. Working with teachers who have a caring attitude is the most influential source for acquiring such an attitude.

How can clinical teachers develop a caring attitude?

In 2008, a review by Sutkin *et al.* found that two-thirds of the important traits in outstanding clinical teachers of medicine are non-cognitive. These traits include relationship skills (e.g. caring attitude), personality type, non-verbal communication and emotional state.

Compared to cognitive traits, these traits are more difficult for teachers to develop. It seems that observing others, reflecting on the experience and then practising these new skills is the way to acquire these skills.

ACTION PLAN

Developing a caring attitude is not something that you will develop overnight. You will need to learn this skill over years of practise.

- Always look for role model teachers to follow.
- Have a mentor.
- Observe how your role model teachers take care of their students, trainees, patients and people working with them.
- Reflect on the experience you learnt.
- Work on replacing your habits and attitudes with the new habits you wished to acquire.
- Practise the skills you learnt and share your experience with your mentor.
- Monitor your progress.

Take-home message

- Showing a caring attitude is a non-cognitive trait teachers seek to develop.
- Developing a caring attitude can be improved through reflection on daily activities and observing role model teachers.

Further reading

Finn K, Chiappa V, Puig A, Hunt DP. How to become a better clinical teacher: a collaborative peer observation process. *Medical Teacher* 2011; **33**: 151–5.

MacDougall J, Drummond MJ. The development of medical teachers: an enquiry into the learning histories of 10 experienced medical teachers. *Medical Education* 2005; **39**: 1213–20.

Pinsky LE, Monson D, Irby DM. How excellent teachers are made: reflecting on success to improve teaching. *Advances in Health Sciences Education: Theory and Practise* 1998; **3**: 207–15.

Sutkin G, Wagner E, Harris I, Schiffer R. What makes a good clinical teacher in medicine? A review of the literature. *Academic Medicine* 2008; **83**: 452–66.

Wright SM, Kern DE, Kolodner K *et al*. Attributes of excellent attending-physician role models. *New England Journal of Medicine* 1998; **339**: 1986–93.

CHAPTER 4

Motivate students and co-workers

… emotional and attitudinal competencies such as self-awareness, self-regulation, motivation, empathy and social skills are required to achieve excellence.

RM Harden *et al.*, 1999

Motivate your students to achieve their goals

Hamza M Abdulghani

CASE SCENARIO

You are an academic staff member in an established medical college that uses a traditional curriculum. Recently, the college has introduced significant changes to the undergraduate curriculum, staff training and development, and the assessment system. You are a clinical teacher responsible for co-ordinating the final clinical year in an ambulatory care unit. You notice that a good number of students are not attending the clinical teaching sessions. You start making enquiries and finding out reasons for their absenteeism, their reply being, 'Our written exam is soon and we have to prepare for it, so we are under pressure; we can attend these clinical sessions after completing the midblock exam.'

This situation has compelled you to think about improving the students' attendance in the clinical sessions, and motivating students to become more interested in learning in a clinical context and achieving their academic goals.

CASE STUDY

The teacher observes that the students do not give due priority to the clinical teaching sessions. In this case, the teacher realizes that the students do not make it a priority to attend clinical teaching sessions as they feel that some sessions do not help them in achieving high marks in their assessment.

Student motivation is a well-researched topic in general education, but less in medical education. The interest in student motivation in medical education has increased, especially in the last decade. Motivation influences students' learning and their performance.

Studies have shown that academic motivation has been shown to be related to increased academic achievement in medical students.

Motivation can be categorized as extrinsic and intrinsic. Extrinsic motivation refers to the act which comes from the external environment, such as parents' pressure on students to obtain high grades and tutors' behaviour. Intrinsic motivation, however, is the desire to do something because it is inherently interesting. Students want to learn as they are curious; they would like to improve, they seek knowledge and skills to learn and learning gives them satisfaction.

The literature surrounding the motivation of students has shown that students respond positively to three elements in most teaching activities: a well-organized course, a teacher who is enthusiastic about his/her teaching, and when teachers show interest and care about their students and their learning.

ACTION PLAN

The following actions may motivate student learning, especially in a clinical context.

- For a clinical rotation, the course to be well organized with regard to its teaching/learning activities, an explicit study guide, logbook, assessment system and grades to be allocated for the students' participation in discussion during clinical teaching sessions are required. Students must know the college's competencies and outcomes.
- Students must be encouraged to actively participate in clinical sessions. Clinical skills should be taught in an engaging way that suits the learning needs of the students.
- When tutors are positive and enthusiastic about their teaching/ learning sessions, students will be motivated to learn. This will be further enhanced when learning occurs in a safe and friendly environment supported by constructive feedback to students.
- Constructive feedback is a strong motivating element in students' learning. Feedback on students' performance should be provided regularly. Clinical teachers should be trained in workshops on how to conduct such sessions.

Take-home message

- There are two types of motivation: intrinsic and extrinsic.
- Students are motivated to achieve their goals when teachers are enthusiastic about their teaching/learning sessions and care for their students.
- To achieve student motivation, teaching activities must be interesting, encouraging and designed in a way that suits students' needs. These sessions should be delivered in a safe environment that enables students to actively participate in the discussion and contribute to learning activities.
- Constructive feedback to students on their performance is an important factor in motivating students.

Further reading

Artino AR, Rochelle JS, Durning SJ. Second-year medical students' motivational beliefs, emotions, and achievement. *Medical Education* 2010; **44**: 1203–12.

Kusurkar RA, Cate TJ, Van Asperen M, Croiset G. Motivation as an independent and a dependent variable in medical education: a review of the literature. *Medical Teacher* 2011; **33**: e242–e262.

Misch DA. Andragogy and medical education: are medical students internally motivated to learn? *Advances in Health Sciences Education* 2002; **7**: 153–60.

University of Southern California. Motivating your students. Available from: http://cet.usc.edu/resources/teaching_learning/docs/teaching_nuggets_docs/2.4_Motivating_your_Students.pdf.

Monitor the progress of your students

Samy A Azer

CASE SCENARIO: THE UNDIAGNOSED CHEST PAIN

Michael Ho is an associate professor of medicine with over 25 years of experience in his discipline. The Faculty of Medicine where he works has recently introduced a mentoring programme and he has been asked to mentor three students. Although he has attended several meetings and a workshop conducted with the purpose of the implementation of the mentor–mentee programme, he does not feel that he will be able to help the three students. This is because he is busy with patient care, clinical teaching, and research work and has no time to spend with these students. Because he did not manage his time and commit himself to mentor the three students, he did not meet regularly with them and failed to provide them with constructive feedback or monitor their progress throughout the academic year.

CASE STUDY

In this case, the teacher did not believe in the value of the mentoring system and his justification was that he was busy with patient care, clinical teaching and research work. As a result, he did not allocate time in his schedule to see these three students on a regular basis and did not commit himself to the mentor–mentee programme, as required. Finding no time to meet with students is not necessarily the only reason for failing to effectively manage the mentor–mentee system as required of him. Other causes may include:

- Lack of the teacher's commitment
- Lack of skills in mentoring and giving feedback

CASE STUDY (continued)

- Lack of staff development in the area of mentoring
- Differences in gender and culture as relative barriers to an effective relationship
- Lack of support mechanisms for mentors
- No rewards allocated for mentors
- No management system established to implement the mentor–mentee process and regularly evaluate its implementation.

What makes a great mentor?

- Committed to his/her mentees.
- Able to create a healthy relationship between mentor and mentees.
- Being knowledgeable and skilful.
- Being responsible and able to listen to the mentees and communicate effectively.
- Ability to motivate and give constructive feedback.
- Believing in the value of the mentoring system and how to use it effectively.

What are the impacts of mentoring?

Benefits for mentees:

- More confident in what they are doing
- Ability to enhance their skills and learning performance
- Ability to achieve their goals.

Benefits for mentors:

- Creating a network of collaboration
- A feeling of satisfaction as a teacher
- Being more able to individualize and disseminate their skills to their mentee.

ACTION PLAN

- Establish staff development programmes in the area of mentoring.
- Ensure that mentors are equipped with the skills required for successful mentoring.

- Train students in workshops about the mentoring system and how mentees should maximize their use of the mentor–mentee system.
- Create a management mechanism that ensures its successful implementation and provide mentors with needed support.
- Establish a reward system for mentors to attract new mentors and maintain high-quality outcomes.

Take-home message

- Medical students' stress has negative effects on their learning and interactions. Working closely with students, supporting them and mentoring their progress could help in resolving such challenges.
- Mentoring students should aim at building them up, enhancing their skills and providing them with pastoral care that enables them to overcome challenges.

Further reading

Buddeberg-Fischer B, Herta K-D. Formal mentoring programmes for medical students and doctors – a review of medical literature. *Medical Teacher* 2006; **28**: 248–57.

Calkins EV, Epstein LC. Models for mentoring students in medicine: implications for student well-being. *Medical Teacher* 1994; **16**: 253–60.

Cook DA, Bahn RS, Menaker R. Speed mentoring: an innovative method to facilitate mentoring relationships. *Medical Teacher* 2010; **32**: 692–4.

Ramani S, Gruppen L, Kachur EK. Twelve tips for developing effective mentors. *Medical Teacher* 2006; **28**: 404–8.

Motivate your co-workers

Masami Tagawa

CASE SCENARIO: A FAREWELL PARTY

It was a farewell party for Professor Akira Nakamura, who has been Professor of Medicine for over 30 years in this medical school, and a prominent gastroenterologist with a major interest in viral hepatitis research. 'I sincerely express my great appreciation to all of my colleagues,' he ends his speech, receiving thunderous applause. The party was crowded with faculty and staff from all departments.

Associate Professor Brown said to his colleague Associate Professor Rubin, 'Fifteen years ago, Akira was the only person who approved my idea and supported my grant application. Without him, I would have given up my research and not attained my current position. He helped further my career too. He recommended me as a fellow of clinical education, because he valued my preference for clinical education over basic research. As you know, I struggled with the balance of research and clinical responsibility, and also with my personal life. I lost my motivation to work at medical school. I am happy working as a director of clerkship now. Michel and Monica, are you crying?' Associate Professor Rubin realized that there were administrative staff standing behind them. 'Yes. Professor Nakamura always introduced us to students and residents as the most important person, and he made us members of departmental meetings. We did our best to live up to his expectations.' Professor Nakamura came over to his colleagues with a smile.

CASE STUDY

Young teachers working in a clinical department have many responsibilities, such as teaching, completing research, clinical work, and performing in competitive and stressful situations. Because of this, people easily lose motivation and burn out. To avoid this, Professor Nakamura provided individual solutions to his younger colleagues, and valued and believed in their abilities. This resulted in encouraging them to achieve their own and the department's objectives. Also, Professor Nakamura forged collaborative relations with administrative staff. People understood that he created a positive culture in his department to encourage his colleagues to work.

Why is it important to motivate your co-workers?

High-quality education is implemented and developed by motivated co-workers. All members of a clinical team, as well as administrative staff, contribute to the educational climate and are potential role models. This determines students' effective learning. Co-workers' behaviour influences students' values and attitudes toward supporting each other and being professionals.

What strategies will you use to motivate your co-workers?

- Offer them challenging opportunities and delegate responsibilities to them.
- Ask for their commitment to a decision they have participated in making.
- Value individual needs and styles, believe in their ability, and provide necessary support for them to fulfil their goals.

ACTION PLAN

To motivate your co-workers, consider the following actions.

- Provide young teachers with challenging opportunities in clinical work, research and education, which are closely related to their own values and personal development. This promotes intrinsic motivation to work.

- Ask for opinions, critiques and alternative plans for team or departmental projects, and positively respond. This increases their feeling of participation and recognition of responsibility as members of a group.
- Communicate your purpose and team goals with co-workers. Once they understand your goals, creativity and motivation to change, let them do things their own way. What you do is observe, provide support in solving challenges, and prevent negative consequences.

Take-home message

- Motivated co-workers will be your best collaborators and supporters.
- To intrinsically motivate your co-workers, nurture a positive environment and promote participation and creativity.

Further reading

Cooke M, Irby DM, O'Brien BC. Leadership for organizational change. In: *Educating physicians. A call for reform of medical school and residency.* London: Jossey-Bass, 2010.

Knowles MS, Holton III EF, Swanson RA. Making things happen by releasing the energy of others. In: *The adult learner.* London: Elsevier, 2005.

Steinert Y. Developing medical educators: a journey, not a destination. In: Swanwick T (ed.) *Understanding medical education.* London: Wiley-Blackwell, 2010.

Have a good sense of humour

Samy A Azer

CASE SCENARIO: MY TEACHER HAS A SENSE OF HUMOUR

Dr Carmichael has been nominated as Teacher of the Year at his university. The top reasons stated by students as to why they nominated him were: 'He made me feel confident, he encouraged me a lot to improve my performance, he had a sense of humour, he enabled me to grow and reach my potential, and he made me love his subject'.

CASE STUDY

Several studies have shown that students prefer teachers who care for and respect them, encourage them and are able to build a professional relationship with them. Teachers who have a sense of humour are usually able to create a healthy environment and encourage students to be open to talk to them and ask for help and support.

Why do teachers need humour?

- Humour helps in creating a safe environment and builds rapport.
- Humour helps in revealing secrets about us.
- Humour helps students to relax and overcome stress, particularly for students who are worried about making mistakes.

ACTION PLAN

- Not everyone can or wants to be funny. Having a sense of humour in your teaching is usually a reflection of self-awareness, culture, and what type of relationship we want to build with others.

- Teachers should genuinely be themselves. However, considering the role of having a sense of humour in minimizing anxiety in the class is vital and should be planned in your teaching.

- Videos of popular comedy programmes/series can be a source for exploration in your teaching sessions.

Take-home message

- Not everyone can be funny. Teachers should genuinely be themselves.

- The use of videos of popular comedy television programmes/ series can be an excellent resource for learning and introducing a sense of humour in clinical teaching.

Further reading

Longhurst M. Physician self-awareness: the neglected insight. *Canadian Medical Association Journal* 1988; **139**: 121–4.

Lopez Nahas V. Humour: a phenomenological study within the context of clinical education. *Nurse Education Today* 1998; **18**: 663–72.

Smith BJ. My thoughts on teaching. *Journal of Veterinary Medical Education* 2009; **36**: 256–9.

CHAPTER 5

Encourage and appreciate diversity

Diversity awareness is best geared towards changing behaviour and informing attitudes through the acquisition of knowledge and skills rather than focusing exclusively upon specific clinical problems.

J Kai *et al.*, 1999

Do not stereotype or speak negatively of others

Roger Strasser

CASE SCENARIO: APPEARANCES CAN BE DECEIVING

You are a third-year medical student in the Emergency Department of Metro Central Hospital. Just after Saturday midnight, an indigenous man who looks quite dishevelled and smells of vomit is brought in by another man. Over the next few minutes, you observe the resident read the note handed over by the patient and then make a rapid assessment of this patient while ignoring the person with him.

After the resident leaves, you learn that this is Mr Tom Williamson, 47-year-old decorator, who was brought in by his neighbour from Smithburg, a rural community of 3000 people, which is over two hours away. In the afternoon, Tom had slipped and fallen, hitting the side of his head on the concrete front steps of his house. Initially, he felt fine but after a couple of hours started feeling unwell and soon began to vomit. His neighbour took Tom to the local doctor who assessed the patient and wrote a note requesting that Mr Williamson have a computed tomography (CT) scan at Metro Central. You learn from the neighbour that Mr Williamson is a respected member of the community who neither smokes nor drinks alcohol.

Meanwhile, the resident's notes state that the patient is most likely an alcoholic and orders some blood tests and plain x-rays.

CASE STUDY

The first question to ask about this scenario is what would the student have learned if she had not stayed with the patient, but had followed the resident? If you were the attending emergency physician that night, you may have recognized the negative stereotyping of the resident or you may have reinforced the

CASE STUDY (continued)

situation by listening only to the resident and not to the patient, his neighbour or the student. It is possible that the student and the resident may learn from this situation that superficial assessment based on negative stereotypes is standard practise, unless you as the clinical teacher challenge the assumptions and model respectful behaviour.

Key teaching points in this scenario include:

- The risk of serious misdiagnosis from superficial assessment based on negative stereotypes
- Acknowledging and respecting the clinical judgement of experienced doctors in the community, including rural physicians
- The importance of acknowledging and listening to individuals who accompany patients
- Respectful behaviour demonstrating cultural competence.

ACTION PLAN

Especially in high-pressure situations, there is a risk of reinforcing negative stereotypes and accepting incomplete superficial assessment. To avoid this situation, it is important that you as a teacher model thoroughness, patience and respect. These are more likely to occur if you take the following actions.

- Take the time to listen and consider the perspectives of each individual including patients, accompanying people/family members, medical students, residents, other learners and staff.
- Question the assumptions which may underlie attitudes expressed and behaviours observed, particularly involving medical learners.
- Demonstrate respect for all people whether they are patients, accompanying people, learners, staff members or medical colleagues.

Take-home message

- The most powerful form of teaching and learning is by example. If you do not stereotype or speak negatively of others, your students will learn from you to do the same.

- All clinical teachers have an obligation to demonstrate respectful professional behaviour towards their patients and health professional colleagues, and to present themselves as positive and effective role models for their students.

Further reading

Hafferty FW. Beyond curriculum reform: confronting medicine's hidden curriculum. *Academic Medicine* 1998; **73**: 403–7.

Kenny NP, Mann KV, MacLeod H. Role modeling in physician's professional formation: reconsidering an essential but untapped educational strategy. *Academic Medicine* 2003; **78**: 1203–10.

5.2

Nurture and encourage diversity

Allyn Walsh

CASE SCENARIO: WE AREN'T ALL THE SAME – THANK GOODNESS

Dr Kowalski volunteered to teach clinical examination skills for the first time. She met her new group of students and arranged the session to start with introductions. She was surprised by how much the student body had changed since her student days. She noticed that some of the students were significantly older, and that there was a different gender balance. Some of the students had been working in other careers prior to medical school. She wondered about other diversity in the group, perhaps less apparent. Proud of her profession and her accomplishments, she had hoped to be a role model to at least some of her students, but wasn't sure how she was going to manage that given how different they seemed from her. As the weekly teaching sessions progressed, she noticed how the students' different contributions to the discussion of clinical scenarios enhanced everyone's understanding. She found that her teaching activities led to her own learning, rather to her surprise.

CASE STUDY

With global migration, many countries have an increasingly diverse population to serve, and also a diverse student body. There are many areas of diversity: sociocultural, ethnic, gender and sexuality, among others. Diversity among students in the health-care professions is an important facet of improving the access of communities of patients to appropriate health care. A diverse student body is thought to facilitate the exchange of information about cultures and value systems and lay the foundation for culture sensitivity.

What are the challenges for teachers in working with students from diverse backgrounds?

There are many challenges to this, one of which is that it can be difficult to be a role model to a student who has important differences from the teacher. Depending on local context, there may be a 'demographic discrepancy' between learners and the teachers who are available to serve as role models. Furthermore, one North American study suggested that some well-esteemed medical teachers were unaware of the difficulties encountered in being a role model and mentor for minority students.

What is the response of students to their diversity?

Several studies have shown that medical students value the opportunity to interact with peers who differ from them, and furthermore this interaction has been shown to promote positive attitudes towards diversity in the learning and social environment. Informal learning environments have the most powerful effect.

How can teachers encourage diversity?

Supporting diverse perspectives and approaches in the teaching setting can enhance students' ability to learn from one another, particularly when applied to clinical cases. Supporting admission programmes that foster diversity (pipeline programmes), as well as other initiatives that foster diversity, can be helpful. At the same time, it is important to recognize that students may benefit from connecting with teachers with similar perspectives and backgrounds for some aspects of role modeling and mentoring.

ACTION PLAN

To encourage diversity in your learners, consider the following actions.

- It is quite possible to be a role model, even when your student is different from you, but it takes open discussion.
- Connect students to other teachers who may share important characteristics with them.

- Where possible, structure student groups and teaching sessions to be as diverse as possible.

- Encourage opportunities for students to interact informally together, for example in study groups.

- Support programmes that aim to foster diversity in the student population.

> Take-home message
>
> - Interactions between students from different backgrounds promote positive attitudes towards diversity. Mentoring and role modelling are also important.

Further reading

Guiton G, Chang MJ, Wilkerson L. Student body diversity: relationship to medical students' experiences and attitudes. *Academic Medicine* 2007; **82**(10 Suppl.): S85–8.

Wright SM, Carrese JA. Serving as a physician role model for a diverse population of medical learners. *Academic Medicine*. 2003; **78**: 623–8.

Seek and encourage understanding of and respect for people of diverse background

Allyn Walsh

CASE SCENARIO: IT'S JUST NORMAL FOR THEM, ISN'T IT?

'Well, I don't know why she doesn't just leave him, if it's really that bad!' said Marcus. Three students were discussing a patient who had just been seen in the clinic. 'He has a serious problem with alcohol and he spends all the money she earns – I wouldn't tolerate that for 5 minutes,' contributed Lillian. Their teacher, Dr Khalid, asked the group what reasons they thought Mrs O would have for staying in what seemed to be such a difficult situation. Marie wondered how acceptable it would be to leave a marriage in Mrs O's family and cultural group. Lillian thought that perhaps this was just a normal situation for them, and that she really didn't expect anything different. Marcus said that he thought she should just move to a new place, without her husband. Dr Khalid asked the group to consider what the barriers might be for Mrs O and how her perspective might be different from theirs. He wondered if he should address Lillian's comment about this being a normal situation for 'them', and wasn't sure how to do so. He decided to let it go.

CASE STUDY

The students in this situation brought their own cultural understandings and biases to Mrs O's situation – as do we all. The challenge is in understanding and accounting for these in the clinical encounter. Dr Khalid encouraged the students to consider Mrs O's perspective and all the factors that she might have to consider. This discussion could have also included appropriate specific ways to explore these with Mrs O in order to provide any help that she might want. Importantly, he also asked them to

CASE STUDY (continued)

look at their own perspectives and assumptions. Understanding that practitioners bring their own cultural preferences and biases to encounters with patients is the first step in dealing with difference.

How can teachers encourage students to become aware of their own cultural assumptions?

Culture is a set of unwritten rules – we take them for granted, so teachers must identify situations where cultural factors are at play and discuss them with students. Students may believe that health-care professionals are culturally neutral and teachers can help through normalizing the reality that we all have assumptions and biases, but must learn to recognize them in order to deal with them appropriately. Gently but appropriately challenging these biases will aid students in this effort.

How can teachers deal with racism, sexism, homophobia and other forms of discrimination when they recognize it?

It is important that teachers explicitly address power relations in the health-care environment. Those in positions with power and privilege tend to be unaware of it and take it for granted, and students in particular often do not feel their power with patients. This can be done through discussions that reveal this power and privilege and appropriately challenging statements or behaviours which stereotype or demean others.

ACTION PLAN

To build an understanding and respect for diversity in your students, consider the following actions.

- Provide opportunities for students to work with patients in a wide variety of contexts, and from diverse backgrounds.
- Be explicit in talking about issues of power and privilege as they arise in the clinical setting.

- Promote student reflection on attitudes, beliefs and biases, to help develop critical self-awareness in professional situations.
- Consider enrolling in staff development sessions dealing with cultural awareness and cultural safety – most people benefit from explicit teaching in this challenging area.

Take-home message

- In an increasingly global and diverse world, teachers can actively encourage students to understand each patient's perspective, as well as the influence of their own culture. By striving themselves to achieve such understanding, they will be excellent role models for their students.

Further reading

Beagan BL. Teaching social and cultural awareness to medical students: 'it's all very nice to talk about it in theory, but ultimately it makes no difference'. *Academic Medicine* 2003; **78**: 605–14.

Kai J, Spencer J, Wilkes M, Gill P. Learning to value ethnic diversity – what, why and how? *Medical Education* 1999; **33**: 616–23.

Creating a culture of equal opportunity

Patricia S Sexton

CASE SCENARIO

The new round of interns arrived on Monday morning at the Internal Medicine Department. Dr BJ Kauffman, chief resident, instructed the junior residents to keep a close eye on the interns and teach them as much as possible. He stated, 'Use the type of instruction you *wish* you had received yourself'. Dr Claire Jacques, a third-year resident, stepped up and said, 'I'll teach them! I'll make sure all the men do the dirty work for once'. Another resident noted, 'Why are there so many foreigners this year? I'm not here to teach English as a second language'. Dr Kauffman calmly reminded the group again that they were role models for the interns and that they should treat them with the same respect that they expect themselves; anything less would be unacceptable. At the next meeting, Dr Kauffman suggested some development programmes be started for both house staff and attending physicians to address respect and personal biases.

CASE STUDY

There are many hierarchies in medicine. Some perceived and others real. In many cases, there are laws mandating that equal opportunity be given to all – regardless of gender, nationality, ethnicity, race or sexual orientation. Subtle disrespect and inequality may remain, however, and are often due to personal bias or experiences from one's past. In this case study, the chief resident has likely either received excellent role modelling in the past or has seen behaviours he doesn't wish to repeat. It is his role not only to help to direct the acquisition of clinical knowledge, but also to help to form behaviours and attitudes. This is the only way the cycle of inequality and disrespect is broken.

Why is equal opportunity necessary in clinical medicine?

Equal opportunity is essential so that all physicians (and other health-care professionals) receive full and appropriate clinical training. This, however, is not the extent of the role it plays. The culture of medicine and the expectations of patients today demand equity. Without diversity, many patient populations never see a health-care provider who is 'like them'. Physicians with varied backgrounds are more likely to serve those who may face inequality, such as the underserved. In the end, creating a culture of equal opportunity is a 'win-win' situation. Colleagues and patients who experience a culture of respect respond accordingly.

What are the characteristics of a culture of equal opportunity in a classroom?

- Teachers who demonstrate respect for students and colleagues instil within all an ethic of treating others the same way.
- Bedside teachers who demonstrate equity on rounds create a competent diverse work environment.
- In an equal opportunity environment, no one feels inferior or discriminated against. This allows the best teaching and learning to occur.

ACTION PLAN

To create a culture of equal opportunity in clinical practise, consider the following actions.

- Use professional development opportunities to discuss personal biases. Bring in people from varied backgrounds to speak with clinicians about the types of prejudice they have experienced.
- Encourage diversity when choosing your team.
- Remember that when teaching individuals, one must first understand the learner's point of view and background.
- Reward teachers who strive to maintain an environment of equality and those who demonstrate this quality for others.
- Review attitude and behaviour expectations before the start of the programme and, if necessary, intervene early if these expectations are not met.

Take-home message

- A culture of equal opportunity allows all learners to be their best and gain equal experience.
- A teacher at any level is a role model, teaching implicitly, as well as an explicit instructor. Ensuring that an equitable environment for learning is an expectation for all allows for the best clinical training and patient care.

Further reading

Cole TR, Goodrich TJ, Gritz ER (eds). *Faculty health in academic medicine*. New York: Humana Press, 2009.

Peterkin AD. *Staying human during residency training*. Toronto: University of Toronto Press, 2008.

Stern DT. *Measuring medical professionalism*. Oxford: Oxford University Press, 2006.

5.5

Maintain positive relationships with students

Allyn Walsh

CASE SCENARIO: A TOUGH JOB

The junior doctors consistently request placements with Dr Cheung, and medical students who work with him regularly nominate him for teaching awards. His students talk about the interest he takes in them, and in their learning, and how he seems to enjoy his clinical work as well as teaching them. Ari, a senior student, was disturbed to receive a mid-placement evaluation with a global rating that was unsatisfactory, along with a request to meet Dr Cheung to discuss the results. Dr Cheung asked Ari his reaction on receiving the evaluation with its written comments, and listened carefully to Ari's explanations. Dr Cheung used the principles of feedback to explain where things were going well, as well as the necessary improvements. Together they planned the next steps that would bring Ari to a satisfactory rating by the end of the placement. Ari left the meeting feeling understood and hopeful that he could turn things around before the end of the placement.

CASE STUDY

In this situation, the teacher did not let his reputation as a popular teacher stand in the way of taking on a difficult task – giving an unsatisfactory rating. In fact, building and maintaining positive relationships with learners allows teachers to do difficult tasks more easily. This student was given an opportunity to explain his ideas, to feel understood, and a partner in the situation.

Despite his unsatisfactory mid-placement rating, the student felt respected by his teacher. Although the student was surprised by the evaluation, the relationship with his teacher gave him a positive outlook, rather than either hostile resistance or hopeless dejection.

Why is it important for teachers to build positive relationships with students?

Teachers have many difficult duties in working with their students; however, when the relationship is one of mutual respect and trust, students will respond better.

In addition, people learn best when they feel safe to take on new challenges, and teachers need to build this sort of safe learning environment.

We know that for students to improve in the clinical setting, they need deliberate, coached practise. It has to be coached in order to be correct. It is very hard to do new things or to change bad habits and a trusted teacher can facilitate these changes.

How does the hierarchy in education affect relationships with students?

Teachers and students have a hierarchical relationship, with teachers having the power to evaluate students and influence their career, more so than the reverse. Different cultures have different gradients to this hierarchy, but in all cases, mutual respect should be demonstrated. It is important to be aware that there can be cultural differences in how this respect is demonstrated in the medical setting.

ACTION PLAN

To maintain positive relationships with students, consider the following actions.

- Take time for introductions in the clinical setting, and use your students' names frequently.
- Ask about their personal learning objectives and needs, and gear teaching towards them when possible.
- Ask the student's perspective on a teaching session or placement first, and listen carefully.
- Use the principles of good feedback (see **Chapter 10**).
- Let your enjoyment of clinical work and teaching show. But when you have a bad day, don't take it out on the students – be positive.

Take-home message

- Demonstrate your interest in each student and their learning needs.
- Listen carefully to students before taking action.

Further reading

Daelmans H, Hoogenbloom J, Donder A *et al.* Effectiveness of clinical rotations as a learning environment for achieving competences. *Medical Teacher* 2004; **26**: 305–12.

Haidet P, Stein H. The role of the student–teacher relationship in the formation of physicians. *Journal of General Internal Medicine* 2006; **21**(S): S16–S20.

CHAPTER 6

Bring a wide range of skills and talents to teaching

What the best college teachers do ... achieve remarkable success in helping their students learn in ways that made a sustained, substantial, and positive influence on how their students think, act and feel. '

K Bain, 2004

Use a wide range of teaching/learning approaches

Jill SM Omori

CASE SCENARIO: BRIDGING THE ATTENTION GAP

Dr Boron felt very confident going into his one-hour lecture on health care maintenance guidelines. He had researched all of the new guidelines and spent several hours putting together a PowerPoint presentation for the students. He felt that this topic was very important for the students and really wanted them to understand it well.

During his lecture, he noticed that many of the students were looking at their phones and had their laptop computers open. Several of the students were also talking to each other and a few were even sleeping. Dr Boron was frustrated by their lack of enthusiasm, especially since he had spent so much time preparing for the talk. He became even more upset after he received his evaluation form for the session which had only mediocre reviews and many suggestions from the students on how to improve the session. At this point, Dr Boron decided that he would decline the next time he was asked to give a lecture.

CASE STUDY

In this case, the teacher was not able to engage his students well and did not take into consideration effective means of teaching this topic. Most learners have a very short attention span and usually will not absorb any new information after 20 minutes in a standard lecture. Could he have broken up his talk using other activities to get the students actively involved in the topic? Could he have used a game to teach the concepts instead of utilizing a traditional lecture?

Today's learners are very experiential and learn best through active engagement and involvement. Alternatives to traditional

CASE STUDY (continued)

lectures include problem-based learning, games, panel discussions, excursions, laboratory experiences, movies and simulations.

The teacher also chose to ignore the evaluations of his session. Instead of being discouraged by the comments, he should have utilized the feedback to improve his future presentations. Just as feedback is important for our learners, it is also vitally important for teachers to continually seek to improve as well.

ACTION PLAN

To keep your students engaged in learning, consider the following actions.

- Try to break up lectures into segments no longer than 20 minutes. When possible, incorporate interactive components as part of the lectures. These can include discussions, videos, role playing, games, reflection or break-out groups.

- Incorporate animations, videos and audio into standard Powerpoint presentations to make them more interesting for your students. However, do not add things into your presentations just to make them more elaborate; rather they should contribute to helping your students understand the material being presented.

- Provide opportunities for your students to apply what they are learning about, soon after they learn it. This will help to solidify their understanding of the topic. For example, you could have them work through cases in groups or as individuals and apply what they just learned to different scenarios.

- When possible, replace traditional lectures with more interactive learning.

- Review feedback from your teaching sessions regularly and use the comments to help make your presentations more effective.

Take-home message

- The current generation of students are experiential learners and need a variety of teaching approaches to maximize their learning.
- Utilize interactive teaching components as much as possible to better engage students in learning.

Further reading

Mann K, Gordon J, MacLeod A. Reflection and reflective practise in health professions education: a systematic review. *Advances in Health Sciences Education: Theory and Practise* 2009; **14**: 595–621.

Norman GR, Schmidt HG. The psychological basis of problem-based learning: a review of the evidence. *Academic Medicine* 1992; **67**: 557–65.

Oblinger DG, Oblinger JL. Educating the net generation. Educause E-book; 2005. Available from www.educause.edu/educatingthenetgen.

Stimulate higher-order thinking skills

Ray Peterson

CASE SCENARIO: BUILDING AND EXTENDING UNDERSTANDING

Joanne is on a clinical psychology student placement in a tertiary hospital and completed an initial assessment of a 68-year-old married woman with metastatic breast cancer. In her assessment, the main issues were the presence of depressive symptoms, such as reduced appetite, feeling sad and tearful most of the time, sleep onset insomnia, poorer concentration, and thoughts and feelings of hopelessness and agitation. It was also noted that the patient has limited social support and was experiencing significant pain issues as a result of progressive disease.

During the discussion with Joanne, the following questions were asked by the preceptor.

- How do we distinguish between grief reactions compared to that of mood disorder (depression)?
- How would you assess pain and symptom control and how much these are impacting on depressed mood and suicidal ideation?
- How would you address the patient's concerns or fears about death and dying, and her worry about the effect of illness on other family members?

CASE STUDY

These preceptor questions promoted higher-order thinking and extended Joanne's understanding linked to other learning to this case. Through these questions, the preceptor develops a deeper understanding of the student's knowledge and skill base, and encourages the student to apply and differentiate the relevant knowledge to the case.

How to ask higher-order thinking skills questions

The preceptor started this process by building on what the student knows. 'What' questions do not usually lead to higher-order thinking alone and testing and extending understanding, as they often only encourage recall of what the person knows. If the conversation stops at this point, no higher-order thinking will have occurred. However, 'what' questions can be a good starting point for subsequent questions which promote higher-order thinking. Starting the thinking process from what the learner knows enables the preceptor to introduce questions which promote higher-order thinking and understanding.

Higher-order thinking questions usually include or imply the 'how' and 'why' words. They are designed to enable the person to comprehend and apply what they know, explore and probe their understanding, differentiate the relevant knowledge, differentiate between alternatives and the implications of decisions to address a situation, and to evaluate and synthesize information from various sources. These questions lead to a shared understanding of what the learner knows, and this may lead to new learning. Some examples of this could be:

- Differentiating: Tell me how …?
- Probing: If this is the case, why …?
- Considering an alternative: What if …?
- Evaluating: How is this different to the previous case of …?
- Synthesis: How do all these clinical findings lead to …?
- Analysis: What is your management plan? How have you come to this decision?

The analysis questions demonstrate the importance of a 'what' question followed by a question that encourages higher-order thinking and understanding.

ACTION PLAN

To stimulate higher-order thinking:

- Ensure you appreciate what the student knows through questions and observation prior to extending their understanding
- Mentally review where the student should be in their learning and what questions may help bridge any gaps

- Rehearse a few higher-order thinking questions which could be used for an upcoming teaching encounter
- Develop a style of non-threatening questioning. This will engage the learner and build positive discussions.

Take-home message

- Higher-order questioning will stimulate higher-order thinking and help the learner develop a better and applied understanding, or better level of performance on the task.
- By stimulating higher-order thinking, both the teacher and the student have better learning and teaching encounters.
- Higher questioning enables the preceptor to guide and focus the learner on the areas that are important.

Further reading

Lake FR, Vickery AW, Ryan G. Teaching on the run tips 7: effective use of questions. *Medical Journal of Australia* 2005; **182**: 126–7.

Present difficult concepts comprehensibly

Damon H Sakai

CASE SCENARIO: A DISCONNECT IN TEACHING AND LEARNING

For the past two weeks, a faculty member noticed that his ward team has been unable to grasp the pharmacology and clinical application of anti-arrhythmic medications despite his efforts to explain. He told them this was a very difficult topic that few are able to grasp. He reviewed the electrochemical effects of each agent in exhaustive detail, including their many effects on action potential duration, sodium current, potassium current, and other ion channels. Despite these efforts, when asked, his students were unable to explain how a given anti-arrhythmic could interrupt a re-entry circuit.

The teacher felt his team was not paying attention. The residents and students felt frustrated. They tried their best to respond to their teacher's questions, but felt the instruction they received was difficult to follow and comprehend. Their motivation to learn the material decreased and they anticipated a poor evaluation at the end of the rotation.

CASE STUDY

In this case, the teacher did not assess the level of knowledge of his students and their learning needs prior to instruction. Was an explanation of the phases of the cardiac action potential and the requirements for the development of a re-entry circuit necessary before covering the different medications? Also, could the teacher simplify the material in a way that would enhance retention? Finally, understanding difficult concepts requires more effort. Could he make the topic more meaningful to increase student motivation to learn?

What strategies will you use to teach a difficult topic?

- Make difficult topics meaningful to motivate student learning.
- Assess student knowledge prior to instruction and adjust instruction to their level.
- Simplify and teach the most important concepts in an organized way.
- Create learning aids to make complex topics more understandable.
- Provide opportunities for application and practise with feedback.

ACTION PLAN

- Share an anecdote to make the topic meaningful and motivate student learning.

  When I started here as a resident I remember responding to a 'code blue' in the telemetry unit we're standing in right now. When I arrived at the patient's bedside, this was the rhythm we identified and the questions we were faced with.

  The teacher shows a rhythm strip to the team and later explains how they were able to save the patient by applying the knowledge they'll be covering in rounds throughout the rotation. He ends his anecdote by saying that while anti-arrhythmics can be a difficult concept to comprehend, it's a topic he loves and he believes his students can learn this topic too and apply its principles to their patients.

- Assess student knowledge of the topic prior to instruction.

  So tell me, how much do you remember about the generation of arrhythmias and how medications are used to reverse them?

- Break down and simplify the topic and focus attention to the most important principles.

  I'm going to focus our learning on the requirements for the creation of re-entry circuits and the phases of the cardiac action potential. For each pharmacologic agent, we'll concentrate on their most important effects on the action potential and not worry about every effect each drug has.

- Synthesize the key information into a learning aid for students to review independently.

I've prepared a pocket card for you that summarizes the major concepts. It also has a table listing the major effects on the action potential for each drug.

- The teacher creates scenarios that students can use to practise what they've learned.

Let's consider our patient, Mrs Jones in room 411. Explain how her arrhythmia could have developed and why we have placed her on this medication. If you aren't sure, I'll help you.

Take-home messages

- Make difficult topics meaningful to motivate student learning.
- Break down and synthesize the information so that your instruction includes the most important information presented in an organized way.

Further reading

Yelon SL. *Powerful principles of instruction*. Philadelphia: Longman Publishers, 1996.

Encourage appropriate evidence to a critique

Zubair Amin

CASE SCENARIO: BETWEEN A ROCK AND A HARD PLACE

'Lectures are boring,' blurted out a student. 'They are useless; tell us what to learn and we can do a better job. I would rather spend the time with the patients,' interjected another. You, as the co-ordinator of a clinical medicine junior clerkship, are in the midst of a regular meeting with the students. One particular concern from the teachers was that there had been a noticeably large number of students missing the lectures lately.

You report back the findings from the discussion with the students to your clinical teachers. You are surprised to hear different views. 'Lectures are essential for teaching; how else can I provide such a large amount of information to the students?' is a typical response. Clinical teachers are adamant that lectures should remain in place. You are reminded that tutorials or self-learning cannot compensate for what the lectures can provide.

Unable to resolve the issue, you raise it to the next level. The head of the department, who is aware of students' non-attendance in the class, informs you that he uses the attendance rate in a lecture as a parameter of quality of teaching among the teachers. His concern is that if you were to abolish or even reduce the number of lecturers he would lose one 'objective' measure of teaching quality that he uses during annual staff review.

CASE STUDY

Here is a potentially contentious situation with a great deal of emotion and little evidence provided to you by the clinical teachers or the head of the department to support one argument over the other. As we practise evidence-based medicine in our daily clinical activities, why can't we implement the same in our clinical teaching?

Before we source evidence, it is imperative that we define the issues as clearly as possible. Here are at least two issues that can be identified: (1) relative efficacy between lectures and self-learning and (2) relationship between attendance in a lecture and the quality of teaching.

Let's try to resolve the first issue through a well-known approach in evidence-based medicine. The acronym PICO stands for Patient, Intervention, Comparator, and Outcome. Using the same framework, we could develop a searchable question. Here the patient is replaced by the 'students', the intervention is 'lecture', comparator is 'self-learning' and outcome is 'performance in clinical examination'. So, the searchable question is 'Is lecture superior to self-learning in improving performance in clinical examination among the students?'.

- Can you formulate a searchable question with the second issue described above?
- What are some other issues in your daily teaching activities that can be answered through an evidence-based approach?
- What search engines or sources (e.g. PubMed) would be useful in finding answers to the questions?

ACTION PLAN

- Identify issues related to education that need evidence to support decision making.
- Try to develop a 'searchable question' that can be answered.
- Identify journals and databases that could be useful in answering the questions.

Take-home message

- Evidence to support sound educational practises is available; like clinical queries they need to be formulated in the right way.
- When formulating educational queries defining the outcome is the key.
- Many reputable professional organizations regularly publish educational guidelines based on best evidence and best practises.

Further reading

Haig A, Dozier M. *Systematic searching for evidence in medical education. BEME Guide 3.* Dundee, UK: Association of Medical Education in Europe, 2003.

Harden RM, Grant J, Hart IR. *Best evidence in medical education. BEME Guide 1.* Dundee, UK: Association of Medical Education in Europe, 1999.

Teach memorably

Richard Kasuya

CASE SCENARIO: THE MEMORABLE TEACHER

Sitting down with a young faculty member over a cup of coffee, our discussion turned to an outstanding teacher that we both had the pleasure of seeing in action.

'She always seems to know exactly what the students need to know at that particular stage of their training, and finds a way to make that material meaningful and simple to understand,' my junior colleague observed.

'Yes,' I agreed. 'And her use of clinical stories, humourous anecdotes, short videos that highlight her points, and opportunities for students to practise what they are learning is always effective and impeccably timed.'

My colleague nodded in agreement. 'Just watching the buzz among the students as they leave her classroom, I can see how they are inspired by her teaching. Even when I run into these students years later, they fondly reminisce about how much she cared about them, and how memorable her teaching was …'.

CASE STUDY

The case above describes a teacher who understands and demonstrates practises that help make teaching memorable to students. The reader might recognize some of the basic ingredients of good teaching within the case, including understanding the needs of students, being able to strategically use novel methods, sharing interesting stories that help add meaningfulness to the material being taught, providing opportunities to practise what is being taught and learned, and clearly communicating passion for the subject matter and a genuine concern for students. Simply put, memorable teaching is the product of thoughtful, student-centred teaching.

What can teachers do to make their teaching more memorable to their students?

- Understand the needs of their students. An appreciation of student goals, needs, expectations and experiences allows teachers to best align their goals, content and methods.

- Simplify complex material. Students appreciate when teachers translate their expert knowledge into a well-organized, easily understood package.

- Use novel methods. Novel methods, such as role-play and debate, can leave a lasting impact on students. These can be especially effective when they help reinforce key points or the core content.

- Strategically share stories. Stories are a very powerful tool to impress meaningfulness and reinforce the importance of the material being taught.

- Supplement slides and oral presentations with video, audio files, or other multimedia tools. Today's students are very comfortable with learning via educational technology. Effective teachers learn how to incorporate these tools into their teaching.

- Be passionate and enthusiastic about the topic and material. These qualities are infectious, and help energize and motivate students to learn.

- Appropriately incorporate humour. Humour is a powerful tool to help bring people closer together. Memorable teachers use humour strategically to connect and energize students.

- Incorporate opportunities for praxis (practise with reflection). Memorable teachers help students solidify their learning through opportunities to practise, reflect and receive feedback.

ACTION PLAN

To teach memorably, consider the following actions.

- Make the effort to learn about your students' experiences and needs.

- Find ways to make the topic and content meaningful to the student.

- Selectively incorporate novel methods, especially if they can help reinforce key points.

- Communicate your passion for your topic, and your desire to see students successfully learn the material.

Take-home message

- Memorable teaching is the product of thoughtful, student-centred teaching.
- One of the primary goals of teaching is for students to be able to recall and appropriately apply what they have learned. Being able to teach memorably is a skill that all teachers should strive to achieve.

Further reading

Ende J. *Theory and practise of teaching medicine*. Philadelphia: American College of Physicians, 2010.

Mann KV. Thinking about learning: implications for principle-based professional education. *Journal of Continuing Education in the Health Professions* 2002; **22**: 69–76.

Model a close doctor–patient relationship

Cindy LK Lam

CASE SCENARIO: AT TIME OF NEED

I just got back to my office after my morning surgery when the telephone rang. It was Mrs Pang whose family I had looked after for more than ten years. She sounded in distress, telling me that her 25-year-old son, Peter, was admitted to the Intensive Care Unit (ICU) after he collapsed at home three days ago. The hospital doctor told them that Peter's blood potassium was dangerously low (1.8 mmol/L) and he suspected thyrotoxicosis. However, Peter refused any further treatment and signed the DAMA (Discharge Against Medical Advice) form. Peter told me over the phone that he could not understand what the hospital doctor told him about his diagnosis and he was very scared because the doctor said that he would be treated with radioactive iodine (RAI). He thought RAI was a kind of radiotherapy that would make him bald. After listening to him, I explained to him that RAI was not radiotherapy and would not lead to hair loss. I assured him that he had the right to refuse a treatment without the need of DAMA. I emphasized the danger of very low blood potassium and that the hospital doctor was trying to help him. Peter then asked, 'Do I have to leave the hospital and come back through the Accident and Emergency Department because I have already signed the DAMA form?'. I told him that all he had to do was to let the hospital doctor know that he no longer wanted to enforce the DAMA.

CASE STUDY

This case illustrated how a close doctor–patient relationship was critical for motivating the patient to accept and adhere to treatment, and how the lack of a trusting doctor relationship could make a patient with a life-threatening condition refuse treatment. Fear and denial made the patient doubt the diagnosis

CASE STUDY (continued)

and management from the doctor. The patient signing the DAMA form was an indication of a complete breakdown of the doctor–patient relationship. It was fortunate that the patient's family called me at their time of need. The close doctor–patient relationship that we had built up over time enabled me to counsel Peter to make a more rational decision.

Why is it important to build up a close doctor–patient relationship?

A close doctor–patient relationship supports the patient to cope with diagnoses and treatments that are unfamiliar to them. It is the best 'drug' of comfort for the patient in distress. It empowers the patient to voice his ideas, concerns, expectations and disagreement without worrying about upsetting the doctor. It facilitates effective communication since both parties know each other, which enables the patient to make informed choices. It also helps to build up the patient's trust of medicine and the health-care system.

What are the characteristics of a close doctor–patient relationship?

- There is mutual trust. The patient trusts that the doctor always acts in his best interest, and the doctor trusts that the patient does not make inappropriate demands.
- There is honest and equal communication.

ACTION PLAN

To build a close doctor–patient relationship:

- Promote continuity of care by the same doctor(s) for each patient
- Build up the relationship over time starting from when the patient is relatively healthy, and strengthen it at times of serious illnesses
- The doctor must be available and willing to help at times of need
- The doctor must listen to the patient's voice with respect and provide the best medical advice at the same time.

Take-home message

A close doctor–patient relationship:

- is built over time and on mutual trust.
- facilitates adherence to treatment.
- is not just being polite and agreeing, but be able to negotiate through disagreement.

Further reading

Balint M. *The doctor, his patient and the illness*, 2nd edn. London: Churchill Livingstone 1986.

Stewart M, Brown JB, Weston WW. The fifth component: enhancing the doctor–patient relationship. In: *Patient-centered medicine: transforming the clinical method*, 2nd edn. Oxford: Radcliffe Publishing, 2003.

Use education in community development

Kun-Long Hung and Yi-Chu Yang

CASE SCENARIO: KEEN FOR COMMUNITY DEVELOPMENT

Students planned a health awareness project for a community, whose residents were mostly elderly. At the very early stage of planning, students enthusiastically discussed and designed the health promotion contents, and they decided the main idea of the project was to promote weight loss. After checking with the teacher, students took the proposal to the community and discussed it with the community leader. Fortunately, the community leader agreed to provide help on the project.

During the execution, students and the teacher met regularly to discuss implementing the plans. However, participation in each session was low, and the students felt frustrated. The teacher blamed it on the marketing strategy, and asked students and the community leader to put more effort into posting posters and sending out flyers. However, the situation stayed the same, and even when people showed up for the weight loss lectures, they were bored and left early. The community leader was frustrated and felt the programme was worthless.

CASE STUDY

In this case, the teacher did not consider that community involvement was the key to a successful health awareness programme in the community, which is why students were not directed to it. At the planning phase, students designed the project without taking opinion from the community, and failed to shape it into a health awareness project that the community could really engage in.

Students should invite the community leaders to participate at the early stages of planning. By interacting with the community, students and the community can easily find out the real issues

CASE STUDY (continued)

the community is facing, and work out feasible solutions. When the community is engaged, it recognizes its own health issues, and a health awareness programme has a better chance of being accepted. Furthermore, it will constantly draw the attention to the topics of community health promotion.

Why is it important to use education in community development?

It is important to get local residents involved. During the process, they will start to think about what they really need, how the plan should be carried out, and why it is important to them. The community is empowered during the process, hence it owns the ability to keep promoting community health itself. Among different approaches of conveying medical information, the engagement of community is the only way to be successful. Through the involvement of the community itself and dialogue in a language the community is familiar with, the acceptance will be improved. In addition, this approach can help understand the actual health needs of the community.

What strategies will you use to achieve your goals?

- Tell your students to allow the community to be involved in the project planning.
- Understand the community needs by listening to the local community.
- Tell your students to make the needs of the community a priority while planning a community health awareness project.
- Encourage your students in designing an evaluation system.

ACTION PLAN

To use education in community development, consider the following actions.

- Make sure your students invite local residents to be involved in the project designing and planning.
- Encourage students to interact with local residents and understand their culture.

> ### Take-home message
>
> - Create a climate that encourages communities to participate in the project. Make them realize that they are the active planners instead of passive participants.
> - Help the residents to engage with the project and invite them to attend every discussion.

Further reading

Issel LM. *Health program planning and evaluation: a practical, systematic approach for community health.* Sudbury, MA: Jones and Bartlett Publishers, 2004.

Zahner SJ, Kaiser B, Kapelke-Dale J. Local partnerships for community assessment and planning. *Journal of Public Health Management and Practise* 2005; **11**: 460–4.

CHAPTER 7

Foster critical thinking

If medical educators state the goal of graduating good critical thinkers with different definitions in mind, it is likely that they will use different methods to screen applicants, apply different curricular approaches to the fostering of critical thinking.

E Krupat *et al.*, 2011

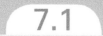

Teach students how to think, not what to think

Ayman A Abdo

CASE SCENARIO: WE ALL ENJOYED LEARNING THROUGH THIS PROCESS

Two first-year medical students, Sarah and Hanan, from two different problem-based learning (PBL) groups were discussing during lunch time how they managed working on this week's PBL case in their groups. The case was about a patient presenting with chest pain. Sarah said, 'We were unable to come up with more hypotheses … we just mentioned stomach problems and heart attack. Our tutor kept asking us what else, what else, but we were unable to think of anything else.'

Hanan immediately responded saying, 'I think this was the most interesting part in the tutorial, we are lucky to have our tutor. She doesn't work with us that way. When we were unable to generate more hypotheses, she asked us to think about the anatomical structures in the chest and the upper abdomen. She asked us to write down these structures starting from the skin and going inward. Once we completed this part she asked us, what could possibly happen to each of these anatomical structures to cause pain? This helped us to come up with over 20 causes. We all enjoyed learning through this process. It helped us to think.'

CASE STUDY

When students are confronted with complex medical problems they usually panic, but once they're encouraged to utilize a system to organize their thinking, the ball starts rolling and they start enjoying the learning process.

Asking questions like 'what else could possibly be the cause of …' is educationally not useful. Asking 'what else' targets memorization of lists rather than thinking processes. A good

CASE STUDY (continued)

teacher should always be able to facilitate students' discussion by using open-ended questions that can engage students and allow them to think about using the knowledge they know from previous sessions in answering new questions.

ACTION PLAN

The following actions may help you in turning your teaching/learning sessions to focus on enhancing students' thinking processes.

- Encourage students to simplify medical problems to their basic roots.
- Encourage students to look for evidence from history and clinical examination for and against each of their hypotheses.
- Recognize common thinking errors during the discussion and facilitate the discussion so that students can recognize what was wrong.
- Help students to be capable of prioritizing the medical problems of a patient in a logical fashion based on seriousness, acuity or patient's concerns.
- Encourage students to think of ethical, social and environmental issues surrounding the case.
- Encourage students to listen and interact with other members of the medical team and receive feedback and input from them.
- Use formative assessment and constructive feedback to enhance students' learning.

Take-home message

- Approaching clinical problems is a challenging mental exercise. Students must develop competencies in logical thinking and problem-solving methods. Helping students develop this skill is one of the most important tasks of a teacher, certainly more important than filling their brains with information that might evaporate soon after.

Further reading

Azer SA. *Navigating problem-based learning.* Australia: Churchill Livingstone, Elsevier Australia, 2008.

Hebert P. *Doing right: a practical guide to ethics for medical trainees and physicians.* Don Mills, Ontario: Oxford Press, 2009.

Muller J, Irby D. Practical teaching: how to lead effective group discussions. *The Clinical Teacher* 2005; **2**: 10–14.

Explore with probing questions

Anthony PS Guerrero

CASE SCENARIO: EVERYONE IS QUIET

Ricky is highly regarded as an intelligent and conscientious student. He presents a detailed discussion on the pathology and histopathology of coronary artery disease. His slides are impeccable and his 15-minute presentation is highly rehearsed and polished. The colleagues and tutor, Dr Grace, are impressed to the point of speechlessness. The presentation ends with the familiar: 'Are there any questions?'. There is silence – followed by 'Okay, who's next?'.

As the students progress in their learning issues and eventually revisit the problem-based case, it is clear that they could not explain the exact mechanisms by which the patient's hypertension, smoking and hyperlipidaemia contributed to the coronary artery disease, or why, at this point, the patient has certain physical and electrocardiogram (ECG) findings. They quietly turn their eyes to Dr Grace, hoping for an expert answer to their questions.

Dr Grace, a relatively new problem-based learning tutor, subsequently consults with the course director. 'So, should I be giving them answers? I usually don't say very much because the presentations seem to be going very well, and they seem to be covering the textbook material.'

CASE STUDY

In this study, the well-meaning tutor and students are missing the point of small-group case-based learning. As detailed as the learning issue presentations may be, it is not clear that any of the students (including the presenters) have understood or assimilated the information in a way that allows them to understand the case better.

ACTION PLAN

To optimally probe the depth and breadth of students' learning, and to evaluate the overall benefit of the group process, consider the following questions. These questions may be useful in any case-based, group learning format, at various stages of medical training.

- During the discussion of an initial problem:
  - 'Are there any other facts or problems that you see in this case?'
  - 'Are there any other hypotheses, or possible mechanisms, for the problem(s) you have identified?'
  - 'Based on that hypothesis, is there any other additional information you would want?'
  - 'Did you have a new hypothesis, based on the additional information you just requested?'
- During discussion of learning issues:
  - 'How would you apply the knowledge you have learned to the patient's presentation?'
  - 'How does the information you've presented relate to what your colleague(s) just presented?'
  - 'It sounds like you have identified a gap in knowledge, and you are wondering if I know the answer. I actually do not know the answer, but how does the group think I would go about finding it? What mechanisms or basic information do you think you need to learn about to help you find the answer?'
  - 'What was the source of your information, and what do you think of the credibility of the source?'
- Addressing group functioning:
  - 'I notice that most (or some) people are quiet. I am wondering what other people are thinking at this point.'
  - 'That was a good clarifying question that you asked your colleague.'
  - 'It seems like there is some disagreement here. Are there any suggestions about how to resolve this?'
  - 'Is there any feedback about today's session: what worked well, and what could have been done better?'

Take-home message

- In small-group clinical teaching, the most important task of the teacher is to ask probing questions that stimulate collaborative learning (so that everyone in the group benefits from the activity), deep understanding, and application of material back to real-life scenarios that one is likely to encounter as a physician. Teachers must engage students in a way that results in meaningful and enjoyable learning.

Further reading

Azer SA. Facilitation of students' discussion in problem-based learning tutorials to create mechanisms: the use of five key questions. *Annals of the Academy of Medicine* 2005; **34**: 492–8.

Norman GR, Schmidt HG. The psychological basis of problem-based learning: a review of the evidence. *Academic Medicine* 1992; **67**: 557–65.

Discuss ideas in an organized way

Anthony PS Guerrero

CASE SCENARIO: THE SHOT-GUN APPROACH

'The patient is a 77-year-old man who lost consciousness and collapsed while tending to his garden. A medically trained bystander was the first to respond, followed by emergency medical personnel.'

After a long pause, one student offers, 'We should rule out a myocardial infarction'.

Another student offers, 'So then we should find out if he's ever had an MI before. Does he take any meds, I wonder?'.

And then another student proposes, 'Maybe it's nothing serious. I fainted once at the mall and people were about to give me CPR'.

Fortunately (remembering advice from the previous year to 'ask probing questions'), the tutor (Dr Grace) asked, 'So how are you coming up with these thoughts and these further questions? Is there some way you're organizing your thinking?'.

With prompts from Dr Grace, the students were able to think about 'the mechanism of losing consciousness' and propose other possible causes, including cardiac problems (that prevent blood from getting to the brain), respiratory problems (that prevent the blood from getting oxygenated) and neurological problems (that directly disrupt functioning of the brain). They then proposed additional history and clinical examination findings that would help to differentiate between these causes.

Subsequently, the students learned that the patient had progressive shortness of breath over the last 8–12 months together with three episodes of brief loss of consciousness over the last 3–4 months. Upon concluding that the cardiovascular causes were more likely than others, they then considered (again, in an organized fashion) whether the problem was in the right or left side of the heart, and whether some of the left-sided problems might include valvular causes, including aortic valve stenosis (which, following an echocardiogram, the patient was ultimately found to have).

CASE STUDY

One key difference between a layperson and a medical professional (in whom lives are entrusted) is the ability to think through and discuss ideas in an organized manner, such that key diagnostic possibilities and management options are thoroughly considered. If one were to approach problems in the 'shot-gun' manner illustrated above or guided only by what comes to mind first or what is most memorable, important facts or possibilities may be completely missed, to the detriment of patients.

ACTION PLAN

When approaching a clinical problem at any stage of medical training, ideas can be discussed according to:

- What are the facts, problems, hypotheses, additional information needed (further history, physical examination and diagnostic tests), and learning issues?
- What is most urgent and most life-threatening?
- What are the mechanisms underlying the presenting problems (from which causative possibilities can then be explored)?
- What, anatomically, are the structures in the region of the body where the problem is occurring?
- What, physiologically, are the processes that could result in the problem (including vascular, infectious, neoplastic, drug-related, inflammatory, collagen-vascular, allergic/autoimmune, traumatic, endocrine, according to the VINDICATE mnemonic, etc.)?
- What are all the organ systems that could be involved (including cardiac, respiratory, urinary, endocrine, haematological, gastrointestinal, locomotor, neurological, etc.)?
- What are all of the biological, clinical, psychological and social impacts of the problem?

When reviewing information researched about a clinical problem, additional organizing principles can include:

- Mechanisms for each of the patient's signs and symptoms
- Coverage of each of the traditional basic sciences (e.g. anatomy, physiology, biochemistry, behavioural science, microbiology, immunology, pathology and pharmacology) that could be relevant.

Take-home message

- Students make the successful transition from layperson to medical professional once they are able to organize their thinking and discuss ideas in an organized way – that ultimately enables safe and thorough care of patients.

Further reading

Guerrero APS. Mechanistic case diagramming: a tool for problem-based learning. *Academic Medicine* 2001; **76**: 385–9.

Kassirer JP. Teaching clinical reasoning: case-based and coached. *Academic Medicine* 2010; **85**: 1118–24.

Help students to focus on key issues

Denise M Dupras

CASE SCENARIO: RECOGNIZING WHAT IS IMPORTANT

You observe a student evaluating a 62-year-old woman who presents complaining of worsening abdominal pain over a period of a week. The patient complains that the pain is low on the left side of the abdomen and associated with occasional bleeding from the rectum. She also complains of subjective fever. You recognize this case as a classic presentation of acute diverticulitis. She has multiple medical problems, including diabetes mellitus, coronary artery disease and stage 2 chronic kidney disease. The student takes a comprehensive history related to the abdominal pain and also of the chronic stable medical issues. He then performs a complete physical examination, including breast and pelvic examination.

The case presentation is organized and covers not only the chief complaint but also detailed discussion of the chronic medical problems. The student then presents his differential for abdominal pain. His differential is extensive and includes appendicitis, pyelonephritis, ischaemic colitis, peptic ulcer disease, renal cell cancer, colon cancer, ovarian cancer, diverticulosis and diverticulitis.

CASE STUDY

In this case, the teacher needs to recognize that the student is collecting comprehensive information, but is unable to recognize the important pieces of information that are consistent with the most likely diagnosis. While he is able to supply a list of things that could cause abdominal pain, he cannot prioritize and incorporate the information from the history and physical examination. The teacher needs to help the student focus on the reason (chief complaint) that the patient is seeking care and the information from the history and physical examination.

Why is it important to help students focus on key issues?

Students first learn to collect information using a script resulting in a comprehensive inventory of signs and symptoms. Focusing on the specific pieces of information that are most important is a critical step in developing a prioritized differential. Focusing on key issues allows the learner to test the information against recognized illness scripts and incorporate the new information into new illness scripts.

What methods will you use to help students focus?

- Identify the key issues or findings in the case.
- Ask what is the most likely diagnosis and why this is most likely.
- For each of the possible diagnoses, ask the student to state what information supports or refutes the diagnosis.

ACTION PLAN

To help your student focus on key issues, consider the following actions.

- Ask the student to list the key issues and why they are key.
- Ask the student to develop a prioritized differential and use the identified case findings to support the differential.
- Ask the student to 'think out loud' to demonstrate the process of synthesizing the information in developing the hypothesis.
- Ask the student to describe a classic case of the diagnosis under consideration when the hypothesized diagnosis is unlikely. Use this to highlight the inconsistencies and guide the student to more likely diagnoses.
- Expose the student to classic presentations of common illnesses to facilitate learning a variety of illness scripts.

Take-home message

- Encourage the student to make explicit the key issues they identify.
- Ask students to 'think out loud' and use the key issues in comparing and contrasting their differential diagnoses.

Further reading

Eva KW. What every teacher needs to know about clinical reasoning. *Medical Education* 2004; **39**: 98–106.

Harasym PH, Tsai TC, Hemmati P. Current trends in developing medical students' critical thinking abilities. *Kaohsiung Journal of Medical Sciences* 2008; **24**: 341–55.

7.5

Train students to think strategically

Denise M Dupras

CASE SCENARIO: ARE THERE OTHER CONDITIONS THAT SHOULD BE CONSIDERED?

A student presents the following case: 'Mr Wilson is a 64-year-old who presents to the office complaining of worsening chest pain, fever and a cough that is productive of a moderate amount of blood-streaked sputum over a period of a week. His vital signs are: pulse is 108 beats per minute, blood pressure 142/84 mmHg, respiratory rate 20, and temperature is 37.9°C. Auscultation of his lungs reveals scattered rhonchi and decreased breath sounds posteriorly on the right. There is pitting oedema in his left leg below the knee. His examination is otherwise normal'. The student tells the teacher, 'I think this patient has pneumonia. I would like to get a chest x-ray and begin him on oral antibiotics'.

CASE STUDY

In this case, the teacher cannot determine if the student has considered any other diagnosis. One way to assess this is to ask, 'Are there other conditions that should be considered in this case?'. If the student has considered other diagnoses, then the teacher should ask why the student considers pneumonia most likely. If the student has no other diagnoses in mind, one approach would be to have the student reflect on what he or she knows about chest anatomy and what else could cause the symptoms. Pneumonia is a condition the student may have seen and has an established illness script of this condition in his memory. The teacher can help the student to develop alternative hypotheses by pointing out inconsistencies in the case with the proposed diagnosis. For instance, asking the student, 'Is a swollen leg common in the setting of pneumonia?' or 'Does the finding of a swollen leg suggest any other diagnosis?'.

A teacher should understand the process of clinical reasoning to be effective in helping students learn this critical skill. Experience with patients provides fertile ground for the student to build new connections between clinical presentations and prior knowledge.

Why is it important to train students to think strategically?

Thinking strategically is critical to clinical reasoning. An important concept in clinical reasoning is the notion of illness scripts. These are constructed from clinical encounters and stored in memory. Their content varies depending on the physician and also on the condition.

The student incorporates the data obtained from the patient, creates a patient representation and then searches for an illness script that matches. This match or mismatch of information informs the next line of investigation to gather additional data searching for defining and discriminating features of the illness. This process is iterative and continues until the student is able to formulate a differential based on the relative matching with the illness scripts the student knows. This process not only drives the diagnostic thinking, but also helps the student to determine which tests are necessary to help differentiate the various possibilities.

What methods will you use to help students think strategically?

- Determine the student's background knowledge of the condition under consideration.
- Ask the student to compare the findings in the case with his or her knowledge of the condition.
- Highlight key findings and ask the student to reflect on this information.
- Model how an 'expert' would approach the problem, be explicit in the key decision points.

ACTION PLAN

To help your students think strategically, consider the following actions.

- Ask the student to compare the developed problem as presented with what the student knows about the disease under consideration.
- Ask about the student's experience and background knowledge of the condition under consideration.
- Ask the student to 'think out loud' through the clinical decision-making process.
- Ask the student to explain how results of suggested tests will inform clinical decision making; for example, 'How will the results of a chest x-ray help you?'.
- Highlight connections between what the student knows about the condition and the clinical presentation to facilitate the learning of new illness scripts when the clinical case cannot be reconciled with a current illness script.

Take-home message

- Begin the learning process with what the student already knows.
- Highlight the connection between what the student knows and the clinical case to facilitate the learning of new illness scripts.

Further reading

Audetat MC, Laurin S. Supervision of clinical reasoning. *Canadian Family Physician* 2010; **56**: e127–e129.

Bowen JL. Education strategies to promote clinical diagnostic reasoning. *New England Journal of Medicine* 2006; **355**: 2217–25.

Pelaccia T, Tardif J, Triby E, Charlin B. An analysis of clinical reasoning through a recent and comprehensive approach: the dual-process theory. *Medical Education Online* 2011; **16**: 5890.

CHAPTER 8

8

Encourage creative work

The teacher who is indeed wise does not bid you to enter the house of his wisdom but rather leads you to the threshold of your mind.

K Gibran, 1883–1931

8.1 Motivate students to create new ideas
8.2 Foster innovations and new approaches
8.3 Show enthusiasm for creative ideas

Motivate students to create new ideas

Tadahiko Kozu

CASE SCENARIO: THINK–PAIR–SHARE

A lecture on fever of unknown origin was being given in a large class session of third-year medical students. During the lecture, the teacher repeatedly provoked students' in-depth active thoughts through open-ended guiding questions.

Then he showed a PowerPoint slide which showed a list of data of a female patient and asked the students, 'What could be the origin of her fever?' and added 'Think independently for two minutes and write down your ideas' (*action A*). There was a ripple of activity as the students wrote their ideas down.

The teacher then said, 'Show your answer to the person next to you, and discuss why you think it is correct. You have three minutes' (*action B*). The room was filled with the noisy buzz of students' conversation.

Three minutes passed. The teacher picked students at random and asked them to share their revised ideas with their classmates after comparison with their neighbouring classmates (*action C*). The responses were active and diverse. The teacher welcomed all different ideas and invited positive evaluation.

CASE STUDY

Problem-based learning (PBL) is undoubtedly a good educational modality to create new ideas through thinking independently, and enhance them by sharing their ideas with fellow students. In this scenario, with all the disadvantages of a large group session, the teacher intentionally used open-ended guiding questions and the 'Think–Pair–Share' technique to stimulate students to create their own ideas.

CASE STUDY (continued)

Spencer Benson's 'Think–Pair–Share' technique consists of 'think' (*action A*), 'pair' (*action B*) and 'share' (*action C*). It has been used in various settings, and will serve effectively in ensuring all students think independently and create their own ideas, even in a large class setting.

Why is it important to motivate students to create new ideas?

Medical education is the preparatory process for tomorrow's doctors. One of the important aptitudes of physicians is thinking independently to create their own ideas and share them with their peers in order to improve or enhance them in team approaches. Such aptitude should be part of the seamless training all through the undergraduate medical education. From the viewpoint of training clinical researchers, continuous nurturing of an intuitive insight into the unknown is imperative.

Problem-based learning is undeniably a good module in motivating the creation of new thoughts. Students may be trained in their problem-solving skills, raising issues and solving problems. However, a large class lecture can also provide an opportunity to stimulate personalized independent thinking and motivate students to create new ideas when the teacher uses guiding questions and the Think–Pair–Share technique.

What strategies will you use to help students create new ideas?

- Train students' self-education through learning in a PBL format.
- Provide the opportunity for metacognition in every learning module.
- In large class sessions, repeatedly offer open-ended guiding questions, or use the Think–Pair–Share technique.

ACTION PLAN

- Stimulate students to think widely and deeply.
- Emphasize the importance of diversity and thinking differently.
- Indicate value in creating new ideas.

- Lead concept formation through schemas and concept maps.
- Lead students to divergence before convergence.
- Ask open-ended guiding questions.
- Apply 'Think–Pair–Share'.
- Feed back positive critiques first to help form students' self-confidence.

> ## Take-home message
>
> - Offer students structured approaches to thinking independently to create their own ideas, and share them with fellow students as a way of metacognition.

Further reading

Brown G, Edmunds S. Lectures. In: Dent JA, Harden RM (eds). *A practical guide for medical teachers*, 3rd edn. Edinburgh: Churchill Livingstone Elsevier, 2009.

Carbone E. Think-pair-share. In: *Teaching large classes: tools and strategies.* Thousand Oaks, CA: Sage Publications, 1998.

Foster innovations and new approaches

Nervana Bayoumy

CASE SCENARIO: WHAT ENGAGES STUDENTS?

'A new group of students today, but no doubt the same dullness,' thought Dr Steve to himself as he made his way to the ward. 'History taking, examination and discussion … these sessions drain me, perhaps I should start being less involved in teaching,' his thoughts continued. Things were not much better with the group of students when they found out that he was their teacher. They all had the same feeling – that it was just going to be quite boring.

Arriving early, Dr Steve had a chance to witness the discussion that went on between the students. They were discussing last night's episode of a popular medical series. They were critiquing the episode, medically of course, what was right, what was implausible and what they would have done. He sensed the enthusiasm and engagement that he longed for in his students. After greeting them, he asked to join in on the discussion and was pleasantly surprised about how much they knew. The rest of the session went a great deal better than it usually did.

Dr Steve and his students agreed to dedicate time in each session to run the same critique for every week's episode. Now, he looks forward to teaching as he finds it enjoyable and stimulating. Also, his students find it engaging as it is much more relevant to them.

CASE STUDY

In this case, Dr Steve found himself caught in the same tedious teaching routine. He even started to contemplate giving up teaching. His students found nothing to engage or encourage them in his sessions. However, the introduction of a new and simple idea to the sessions made a significant difference. The students now look forward to his sessions as they are

CASE STUDY (continued)

more relevant to them. They are motivated and challenged. Furthermore, Dr Steve finds the sessions exciting and enjoyable. He plans to frequently search and implement new approaches, with the help of his students.

Why is it important to foster innovations and new approaches?

New ideas and new methods are essential in teaching for both teacher and students. They help create an interesting and engaging environment. Fostering innovations and new approaches provides a welcomed and much needed challenge in teaching.

What strategies will you use to achieve your goals?

- Consult with students on several new ideas and methods and search the literature for inspiration.
- Study the practicality of these ideas and decide on one or two new approaches to be implemented.
- Assess when is the appropriate time for their implementation.
- Initially, introduce on a small scale.
- Seek feedback from your students.
- Evaluate the success and areas of improvement of the new method/ idea.

ACTION PLAN

To foster innovation and new approaches, consider the following actions.

- Be vigilant for signs of boredom and disengagement from students.
- Observe significant changes in student behaviour and their environment. What appeals to them now most probably would not in five years' time.
- Provide students with an open and safe environment to express their true feelings and opinions.
- Regularly search the literature for new ideas and approaches.

> ## Take-home message
>
> - Innovation and new approaches will protect against senility in teaching.
> - The challenge of introducing new ideas and methods is essential to stimulate both teachers and students.

Further reading

Hartley P, Woods A, Pill M. *Enhancing teaching in higher education: new approaches for improving student learning.* London: Routledge, 2005.

Light C, Calkins S, Cox R. *Learning and teaching in higher education: the reflective professional.* London: Sage Publications Ltd, 2009.

Show enthusiasm for creative ideas

Badran Alomar and Samy A Azer

CASE SCENARIO: I CAN SEE HIS ENTHUSIASM

Sharon Brown, a third-year medical student, comes in to see her teacher with two other students, Lilly and James, to discuss their research project. Sharon has a new idea for the project, completely different from those suggested by her teacher. Although she is not sure that Lilly and James will support her idea, she continues explaining some details to them. The idea is not finalized and there are gaps in it as well as several unanswered questions. However, the teacher shows passion about the idea and suggests that continuing work on the project will fill the gaps.

The next day, the three of them come up with solutions and creative ideas to add to Sharon's proposal. She remembers how the enthusiasm of her teacher about his support motivated the three of them to work on the idea and achieve tangible outcomes.

CASE STUDY

In this case, the teacher shows enthusiastic and unconditional support for an idea in its early stages. He is flexible and very willing not to impose his own ideas on his students. Such support and enthusiasm about an idea, even when the idea is not fully explored, allowed the students to think, research, create and find solutions.

What does research tell us about the impact of a teacher's enthusiasm?

A teacher's enthusiasm helps students to:

- See learning as an enjoyable experience
- Retain information

- Love the subject taught
- Perform better in their examinations
- Set a positive tone in a group setting.

Can enthusiasm be measured?

Though enthusiasm can be considered an innate characteristic, some work in the literature found that outstanding lecturers when compared to novice lecturers tend to show more:

- Vocalization of words
- Eye contact
- Posture/body language
- Movement as they give their lecture
- Facial expression.

ACTION PLAN

Showing enthusiasm for what you are doing changes people around you and engages them.

- Watch a video recording of one of your lectures or a small group discussion you are facilitating. How do you see yourself? Observe your eye contact, vocalizing or emphasizing a particular issue, as well as your facial expression, movement and body language. How do you see the engagement of the students with you in these videos?
- Enthusiasm is a reflection of your state of mind, experience and accumulated skills. Reflection enhances these components and helps you to show enthusiasm in your teaching. Start your reflection today.
- Show enthusiasm, not just for your own work but also be enthusiastic about the work of others around you.

Take-home message

- Your ability to show enthusiasm in your teaching sessions will make a significant impact on your students.
- Without enthusiasm, your ability to engage your students will be lessened.

Further reading

Bauer CF. What students think: college students describe their higher school chemistry class. *The Science Teacher* 2002; **60**: 52–5.

Bettencourt EM, Gillett MH, Hull RE. Effects of teacher enthusiasm training on task behavior and achievement. *American Educational Research Journal* 1983; **20**: 435–50.

CHAPTER 9

Place strong emphasis on teamwork

Coming together is a beginning
Keeping together is progress …
Working together is success.

H Ford, 1863–1947

Encourage students to work in groups

Michelle McLean

CASE SCENARIO: IT TAKES AT LEAST ONE OTHER PERSON TO SELF-ASSESS ACCURATELY

As the co-ordinator of a clinical clerkship, you notice that Ahmed has excellent physical examination skills, but his clinical knowledge is below par. His grades should be higher as he is keen and diligent. You discuss how he might improve in the forthcoming examinations. Ahmed states that he finds it difficult to pinpoint his deficiencies.

While Ahmed practises his physical examination skills with colleagues, he studies alone as he lives at home and his colleagues are in the hostel. You suggest that he organizes a study group that meets after hours. You explain to Ahmed that by discussing topics with colleagues, he will be able to identify deficiencies and iron out misunderstandings.

A few weeks later, Ahmed reports back, beaming. *Why had he not arranged a study group earlier?* He tells you that when he explains something in his own words to his study friends and they validate what he has said, then he knows that he truly understands.

CASE STUDY

Ahmed is clearly experiencing difficulty identifying gaps in his knowledge. His clinical skills are excellent as he practises with colleagues and can compare his performance with theirs. By studying alone, Ahmed is finding it difficult to self-assess. By studying alone, he is not really able to check his understanding. He comes to realize the value of group work.

Why is it important to get students to work in a group?

Self-assessment is not easy. The literature states that those who are least able are also least able to self-assess, i.e. students who fare poorly are probably not able to identify their deficiencies. Group work allows students to gauge their performance relative to that of their peers, i.e. have a reference point. At least one other person is therefore required to help us self-assess accurately.

What strategies will you use to achieve your goal?

- Make learners aware of the need for group work as part of ongoing professional development and improvement.
- Create a culture that allows for reflection and self-assessment (which requires feedback) among learners.
- Develop in learners the skills of giving and receiving feedback (for knowledge, skills and even professional behaviour).

ACTION PLAN

To encourage learners to work in a group, consider the following actions.

- Use group work in your teaching practise. Particularly in the early years, using team-based learning in at least one section of your curriculum will clearly demonstrate the benefits of collaborative effort in learning.
- Incorporate sessions involving peer and self-assessment. Video recordings of students learning communication or physical examination skills are useful in this regard.
- Be a role model in terms of what it means to be a member of a functional and efficient team or group.

Take-home message

- Identifying one's strengths and weaknesses is not easy. Working in a group is one way of checking that you are on track. As a teacher, it is our responsibility to help students to become better at self-assessment, to identify their strengths and weaknesses. We can do this by role-modelling the process, by serving as mentors and by guiding learners through the process of professional development. Inculcate the habit of constantly seeking feedback. Encouraging students to work in groups and to solicit feedback from peers are two strategies to assist learners to gauge the level of their professional competencies.

Further reading

Eva KW, Regher G. Knowing when to look it up: a new conception of self-assessment ability. *Academic Medicine* 2007; **82**: S81–S84.

Parmalee DX, Michaelsen LK. Twelve tips for doing effective team-based learning. *Medical Teacher* 2010; **32**: 118–22.

Encourage collaborative and interprofessional learning

Saad Bindawas

At a 900-bed university hospital, the new dean, who is also director of the Medical and Health Sciences School of the hospital, started receiving complaints from patients and their families about the quality of care, safety and service. The dean believed that these complaints have value and wanted to use them to improve.

Therefore, he assigned a task force to investigate these concerns and to suggest solutions to improve the quality of care and education. The preliminary findings of the task force revealed that the main reason for these concerns was the lack of mutual collaboration between the members of the health-care team and no interprofessional learning culture in the hospital.

In order to deliver high-quality care efficiently and improve the health professional students' learning, the task force recommended the implementation of a method that promotes and fosters interprofessional teamwork and collaboration. Academic and clinical teachers from different health professions (medicine, nursing, physical therapy, pharmacy, dietetics, clinical psychology, speech and language, pathology, dental and many others) were called for a meeting to support a strategy of implementing interprofessional education (IPE).

CASE STUDY

In this case, the university hospital, as any other academic health centre, faces the challenge of providing cutting-edge health care, education and research. The task force found that there were dysfunctional professional relationships (between physicians, nurses, physical therapists, pharmacists and many more), which led

CASE STUDY (continued)

to decreasing efficiency and co-ordination, and ultimately worsened patient and health outcomes. Health professional students need to be introduced to IPE at different stages of the curriculum during their first year, senior year, or during their clinical years.

Why should teachers encourage interprofessional education?

There is substantial evidence that IPE is believed to enhance learners' understanding of other professions' roles and responsibilities, while fostering mutual respect and understanding between members of the health-care team. Studies also showed that health professional students who learn together at the beginning of and throughout their training would be better prepared to deliver an integrated model of collaborative clinical care after entering practise. Such a model of practise is believed to improve quality, reduce errors, and increase satisfaction.

How can a culture of interprofessional education be developed?

- Design a development programme directed towards all academic and clinical teachers from different disciplines, focusing on educational competencies, components and activities for successful IPE.
- Ensure that all students have the basic knowledge, attitudes and skills to learn and work collaboratively.
- Use any possible learning location to implement IPE such as classroom, simulation centre, hospital or clinical settings, laboratory or other learning environment.
- Evaluate multiple aspects of students' interprofessional learning and the impact of this collaborative practise on the institutional culture and health outcomes.
- Publish and disseminate the results of the evaluation(s) and any IPE material or method used to build an evidence base for IPE.

ACTION PLAN

To establish interprofessional education and collaborative practise, consider the following actions.

- For an effective IPE experience that triggers learning, collaborate with other academic and clinical teachers in creating cases, incidents or authored scenarios drawn from past experience.

- Start by encouraging interprofessional learning in undergraduate courses, especially during the preclinical years (e.g. anatomy, pathophysiology, pharmacology, etc.).

- During the clinical years, teach selected curricular topics that encourage interprofessional learning and empower students from different health professions to work together in caring for patients with chronic or acute conditions, or with special patient populations (e.g. patients with HIV/AIDS, mental illness, disabilities, etc.).

Take-home message

- Interprofessional education occurs when two or more professions learn with, from and about each other to improve collaboration and the quality of care.
- Medical and health professional students who are trained in an IPE environment are more likely to work effectively together when they graduate.

Further reading

Interprofessional Education Collaborative Expert Panel. *Core competencies for interprofessional collaborative practise: report of an expert panel.* Washington, DC, 2011. Available from: www.aacn.nche.edu/education-resources/IPECReport.pdf.

Jensen G, Harvan R (eds). *Leadership in interprofessional health education.* Sudbury, MA: Jones and Bartlett Publishers, 2009.

World Health Organization. *Framework for action on interprofessional education and collaborative practise.* Geneva: WHO, 2010. Available from: http://whqlibdoc.who.int/hq/2010/WHO_HRH_HPN_10.3_eng.pdf.

Encourage links at national and international levels in education

Peter Dieter

CASE SCENARIO: WHEN BUILDING INTERNATIONAL LINKS IS IGNORED

In a faculty board meeting, members of the Students' Council complained about the lack of an offer of support from the deanery to facilitate and support links on national and international levels. The dean apologized, but stated that at present the medical school was not able to provide financial or personal resources: all faculty resources were needed for an excellence programme in medical research which would (assuming a positive decision) provide millions in grant money. He asked the faculty members to volunteer to help, but none of the faculty members was willing to do so. After the faculty board meeting, students from the Students' Council decided to protest with a public demonstration and, if necessary, go on strike.

CASE STUDY

In this scenario, the general question is raised about the assignment of a medical school and the importance of medical education, medical research and patient care at the institution. In public rankings, the recognition of a medical school (university) is done primarily by research, followed by patient care and lastly by medical education. Many deaneries follow these criteria. In contrast, most of the students and a number of staff would like to focus more intensely on medical education, including national/international links. However, the deanery offers no financial and personal support for staff in all aspects of education except research, and very often there are even disadvantages associated with staff focusing on education.

How do we change the policy of the deanery?

- Identify students and staff, including 'friends' of the deanery, who are motivated to focus on medical education and national/international links.

- Identify medical schools nationally and internationally with 'good links' to the deanery with a good reputation (in medical education, research and/or patient care) and which are interested in national/international links and partners.

- Create a climate of motivation and enthusiasm.

ACTION PLAN

- To identify a leader and manager for a faculty development programme on 'Implementation of national/international links in medical education, research and patient care'.

- To assemble students, staff and external partners who are interested in/motivated by the programme.

- To identify medical schools nationally/internationally that are willing to co-operate (partner schools).

- To prepare a proposal for the implementation of the programme with a focus on the benefit and national/international recognition for the medical school and deanery.

- In medical education, the proposal must include:

  – semester/study: bilateral exchange of students' year including approval of course achievement by learning/assessment agreements and/or credit systems with partner schools

  – possible reform of the curriculum with free time periods/elective terms to encourage students to spend the elective term in another school overseas/same country (education, research, patient care)

  – clinical observerships: bilateral exchange of students including approval of course achievement with partner schools

  – clinical clerkships: bilateral exchange of students including approval of within-course achievement with partner schools.

Take-home message

- The medical school must formulate a policy for national and international collaboration/links with other institutions, including the approval of courses.
- The medical school must facilitate national and international exchange of students (and staff) and provide appropriate resources.

Further reading

Basic Medical Education. *WFME global standards for quality improvement.* Available from: www3.sund.ku.dk/Activities/WFME%20 Standard%20Documents%20and%20translations/WFME%20 Standard.pdf.

Dieter PE. A faculty development program can result in an improvement of the quality and output in medical education, basic sciences and clinical research and patient care. *Medical Teacher* 2009; **31**: 655–9.

Drain PK, Primack A, Hunt DD *et al.* Global health in medical education: a call for more training and opportunities. *Academic Medicine* 2007; **82**: 226–30.

CHAPTER 10

Provide positive feedback

… negative or constructive feedback is often avoided by clinical teachers, but this is vital to ensure good patient care.

S Ramani and S Leinster, 2008

Listen to your students and discover their educational needs

Susan J Hawken

CASE SCENARIO: WHAT WOULD YOU LIKE TO EXPLORE FROM THIS INTERACTION?

I have been talking to a female patient about the need for a sensitive examination, offering information, gaining consent for the examination and for a medical student to observe. The intimate examination takes place and after the patient has left I ask my student, 'What would you like to explore about this interaction?'.

In this case scenario, I could have many agendas as the clinician teacher, e.g. teaching about the importance of cervical screening or the patient's vulnerability. However, what is more learner-centred is finding out what the student wishes to know.

CASE STUDY

I could utilize some well-researched models to discover my student's educational needs around this interaction. The one-minute preceptor model suggests you obtain a commitment from the learner about what is going on, probe for underlying reasons, teach a general principle, provide positive feedback and correct errors. It is a time-efficient way of teaching at the bedside and has been shown to be more effective than other more traditional teaching modes. The SNAPPS model (summarize, narrow down, analyse, probe and plan) is useful for more advanced learners to explore their underlying clinical reasoning more fully.

How can I listen more to my students?

However, before employing a teaching model, it is important to assess a learner's needs quickly by asking good questions and having the ability to listen and observe. Assessing the level of the learner and listening without interruption have been shown to promote more effective teaching. It may be that the male student is still processing his feelings around observing his first sensitive examination or he may have seen many and be more interested in the impact of the new HPV (human papillomavirus) vaccine on cervical cancer rates. Giving time for the student to reflect and then state what they did not understand ensures you are meeting the real needs of the learner.

Taking a wider view, it can be considered that listening to students is part of a reflective process and that teachers need such information to improve their practise. Useful information may come from this interaction that may inform curriculum development. It is helpful to have both formal and informal systems in which to gather information from students. It is important to utilize skilled questioning and employ active listening so that everyone is heard and all needs are addressed. It is further imperative that you build a culture of trust and develop a relaxed ambience. It is important to note that the context of the learning environment often fluctuates with different students, time changes and different settings. Other methods to collect information include focus groups (preferably through bringing in an independent facilitator) or developing a critical incident questionnaire. Rapid feedback through listening is likely to be timely and contextually relevant and can meet the needs of students and changes can be integrated into the next teaching opportunity. The aim behind good listening is to improve your teaching, but also enable your students to achieve their educational goals.

ACTION PLAN

To create a climate of reflection and promote listening in your teaching practise, consider the following action points.

- Always ask what the student/s wish to explore about the learning interaction they have been involved in and listen attentively.
- Show students that you are receptive to their feedback and that you are able to constructively respond to their ideas.
- Be aware that students come from diverse backgrounds and have different capabilities and needs.
- Create different ways for students to express themselves:
  - anonymous questionnaires can be a safe way to gather information but do not allow you to follow up concerns or probe deeper into issues that may be raised

- interviews and focus groups allow for more in-depth discussion, but students may feel unsafe and thus censor their ideas
- independent reviewers may be useful, but also may not have the contextual understanding of the learning environment in which you are teaching.

- It may be prudent to use multiple ways of listening to your students to triangulate the issues.

- It is useful to have a suggestion box or ask students to keep a journal about their learning experiences.

- Employ systems for synthesizing and enabling students' perspectives and opinions.

- Have systems in place for reflection especially when encountering student disagreement.

Take-home message

- Good listening improves your teaching and allows you to meet the needs of your students and also enables them to attain their educational goals. To enhance the process of listening requires careful questioning and active participation in a trusting, reflective and receptive teaching and learning environment.

Further reading

Irby DM, Wilkerson L. Teaching when time is limited. *British Medical Journal* 2008; **336**: 384–7.

Ottolini MC, Ozuah PO, Mirza N, Greenberg LW. Student perceptions of effectiveness of the eight step preceptor (ESP) model in the ambulatory setting. *Teaching and Learning in Medicine* 2010; **22**: 97–101.

Teherani A, O'Sullivan P, Aagaard EM *et al.* Student perceptions of the one minute preceptor and traditional preceptor models. *Medical Teacher* 2007; **29**: 323–7.

Wolpaw TM, Wolpaw DR, Papp KK. SNAPPS: a learner-centered model for outpatient education. *Academic Medicine* 2003; **78**: 893–8.

Value students, never belittle

Anthony PS Guerrero

CASE SCENARIO: THE INFAMOUS DR STERN

Dr Stern is the ultimate autocratic teacher, infamous for his 'Stern rounds', where prepared students would be 'grilled' with questions until they reached the limits of their knowledge, and unprepared students would be publicly belittled.

One day, Dr Stern meets with the one person in the physician hierarchy who is higher than he is (though slightly less senior) for an annual performance review. 'You're a very knowledgeable and highly regarded attending physician who has trained generations of successful practitioners, but is there any way you can tone down your gruffness? The last thing I want is a harassment or retaliation complaint from one of our students, and I'm sure you don't want that either.'

Dr Stern's face turns red. 'I know what I'm doing. How else are you supposed to be motivated to learn? Are you seriously listening to feedback from people who don't have any clue yet what it means to be a doctor?'

The supervisor responds. 'I used to feel the same way until recently. I didn't think that the new generation of doctors could ever be as good as we were, until my mother had a femur fracture on the first day of the year, when all consultants were either on holiday or managing other crises. The young orthopaedic registrar performed the operation and the outcomes were outstanding. The registrar had excellent technical skills and excellent communication skills, which I knew I was deficient in when I was at that stage of my career. This situation changed the way I view and interact with my students. Do you realize that these students that you're gruff with and whom you humiliate are the ones who'll be taking care of you and your loved ones in the future?'

CASE STUDY

Students will learn and care for patients most effectively if they feel encouraged, supported and respected at all times in their training, even when receiving feedback. Devalued, belittled and intimidated students will not be able to effectively engage in the group processes necessary for meaningful learning or develop the critical and creative thinking abilities that are needed in health care. They may even become afraid to raise concerns even when a patient's life may be in danger. Finally, if students perceive that they have not been treated respectfully, they will be at risk of devaluing or belittling their own patients. While it is important to hold students accountable to high standards of competence and professionalism, it is not necessary to belittle or humiliate them in the process.

ACTION PLAN

If our goal in medicine is to treat everyone – including our students – with respect, we should constantly ask ourselves:

- How would I feel if I were on the receiving end of my interactions with students?
- What kind of interpersonal values do I want to instill in those who will at some point take care of my loved ones or me in the future?
- Am I a good role model for how my students should treat their colleagues?
- How am I likely to be remembered by the students who will one day be my colleagues?

Take-home message

- Students will optimally learn the competencies of professionalism and effective interpersonal and communication skills if they see effective role models in their teachers. Previously accepted 'hazing rituals' that institutionalized and trans-generationally transmitted mistreatment of students are antithetical to the safe and collaborative practise of medicine.

Further reading

Antonelli MA. Professionalism in the teacher–learner relationship in medical schools: mistreatment. *Hawaii Medical Journal* 2009; **68**: 88–9. Available from: www.hawaiimedicaljournal.org/68.04.088.htm.

Heru AM. Using role playing to increase residents' awareness of medical student mistreatment. *Academic Medicine* 2003; **78**: 35–8.

Provide constructive feedback and formative assessment

Ray Peterson

CASE SCENARIO: YOU NEED TO BECOME A LITTLE SMOOTHER

Jane, a physiotherapy student, had just completed the physical examination of a knee on a real patient. On review, Jane believed she remembered most of the questions to ask and completed the assessment within the required time, but felt 'bad' that the patient appeared to be in pain throughout the assessment, and was scared to 'push' the patient to their maximum range of movement.

Her preceptor responded: 'I think that you completed the basic knee assessment within the required time, which can be a challenge for many students. You introduced yourself well, positioned the patient comfortably and your manual handling of the knee was very supportive. When assessing knee range of movement for someone who has just had a total knee replacement, keep in mind that the patient will experience some surgical wound pain despite the patient having analgesics prior to physiotherapy. It is important that you educate and reassure the patient that there will be some pain with moving the knee, but it is important that they push their range as much as possible, to avoid having a stiff knee in the long term. You also used observation to assess the range of movement; however, it is extremely important to use a goniometer in this population, as it is much more accurate and reliable.'

'Two areas need improvement. (1) Educating the patient about what you are going to be assessing and why, which would involve explaining your assessment in simple lay language in a few sentences. (2) Accurately assess and record knee joint range of movement using a goniometer.'

The teacher then went on to demonstrate the level required for a third-year physiotherapy student.

'I know you were nervous this time when talking to this patient, but you need to become a little smoother and more comfortable when talking to the patients. I will be reviewing a patient this afternoon and I will try and demonstrate some of these communication elements for you.'

CASE STUDY

This scenario combines the use of feedback and assessment of performance to guide learning. The preceptor built on the student's self-assessment and identified areas for the student to work on and a plan forward. Formative assessment was integrated in that the student was given guidance on what needs to be achieved. The teacher contributed to the plan by demonstrating the communication skills required.

Formative assessment and the associated feedback are designed to help the learner improve. Without this assessment, the student is unable to progress and meet the expected levels of performance.

ACTION PLAN

- An environment of mutual respect and rapport will ensure that formative assessment and feedback are delivered constructively.

- Asking the student to assess their learning and clinical performance provides a starting point for constructive feedback.

- Reinforce positive outcomes and areas where the student has met the assessment levels.

- Explain the required level of performance, as expectations for a novice student, final-year student and early-career practitioner are different. The student may not know these different levels of performance. The preceptor should understand these different expectation levels as well.

- Students expect criticism as their form of assessment and feedback, so it is important to highlight the student's strengths and further refinements that can be made. This can include extending the skills of high-performing students.

> ### Take-home message
>
> - Constructive feedback and formative assessment are integrated and designed to help the learner improve.
> - Formative assessment should be delivered in a setting of professional respect.
> - Formative assessment should provide the learner with the levels of performance expected and guides further learning.

Further reading

Archer JC. State of the science in health professional education: effective feedback. *Medical Education* 2010; **44**: 101–8.

Rushton A. Formative assessment: a key to deep learning? *Medical Teacher* 2005; **27**: 509–13.

Help and support your students to grow

Samy A Azer and Fawaz Al-hussain

CASE SCENARIO: MY NEW MENTOR HELPED ME TO MAKE A DIFFERENCE

Lee Richard, a fourth-year medical student, appears to be uninterested in attending the paediatric rounds and bedside teaching sessions. Her absence was reported to the clinical dean, Dr Albert Beckman, who asked his personal assistant to ask Lee to come and see him. Dr Beckman asked the Medical Education Department to provide him with more information about the performance of Lee in previous blocks/modules. After meeting with Lee and her mentor, Dr Beckman felt that Lee might need to have a new mentor to work closely with her. The new mentor, Dr Allan Mark, was able to provide excellent support to Lee. His motivation and continuous support helped Lee to change her attitude and become more focused and committed to the teaching/learning sessions in paediatrics. She also started to enjoy working with children in the outpatient clinic, taking medical history from parents, examining patients, and presenting her findings to her small group during the rounds.

CASE STUDY

This case highlights the role of teachers in supporting students and working with them to overcome any learning challenges. Identifying these students and referring them to good teachers usually helps in providing such care at an early stage of facing learning challenges. In 1997, Ende suggested that all clinical teachers should ask the following questions prior to a teaching encounter and they should be prepared to answer these questions.

- What do you hope to accomplish?
- What is your point of view?

CASE STUDY (continued)

- How will your learners be engaged?
- How will you meet the needs of each learner?
- How will your teaching/learning sessions be organized?
- Are your teaching/learning sessions successful? How do you know?

What are the barriers that can stop students growing and achieving their potential?

- Not addressing their teaching and learning needs.
- Demotivation.
- Teachers not engaging students or giving them the opportunity to take the lead.
- Students focusing on factual knowledge rather than thinking critically.
- Teachers not providing their students with constructive feedback.
- The teaching and learning environment is unhealthy and not allowing students to express their views, and learn from their mistakes.

How can teachers help their students grow?

- Encourage them to focus on their purpose.
- Support them in taking on an active role in the teaching/learning sessions.
- Help them in refining their goals and objectives.
- Provide them with constructive feedback.
- Create a healthy environment where students can express their views even if they are wrong.
- Engage them in reflecting on what they have learnt.

ACTION PLAN

To help your students grow:

- From the beginning, assure your students that you are available and will be happy to answer their queries and support their learning

- Work on creating a healthy teaching/learning environment and build a professional student–teacher relationship
- Always ask students what they wish to explore about the learning interaction and listen attentively to them
- Give constructive feedback to your students and ask them to give you feedback on your teaching and learning
- Encourage students to reflect on their learning and how to handle challenging situations.

Take-home message

- One of the main roles of a teacher is to help students to grow and achieve their potential.
- A good teacher is able to attract students to his/her discipline and make them grow through knowledge, skills and the professional attitude they will acquire.

Further reading

Ende J. What if Osler were one of us? Inpatient teaching today. *Journal of General Internal Medicine* 1997; **12** (Suppl. 2): S41–8.

Ho MT, Tani M. What medical students value from their teachers. *Australian Health Review* 2007; **31**: 358–61.

Teach students how to monitor their own progress

Zubair Amin

CASE SCENARIO: LEARNING TO MONITOR OWN LEARNING

You are in charge of mentoring a group of students. You have been assigned to six students from the third year, which is their first clinical year. You have met with them a few times over the last couple of months. The group consists of a mix of students with varying levels of capabilities and prior examination results. As you interact with the students, you notice that there is one student who is really outstanding academically and truly motivated. However, you have also received reports from the education directors of various postings that two of the students are 'weak'. In one of the regular meetings, the group requests your help in their learning and clinical training. One of the students comments, 'We don't know whether we are on the right track'. A second student shares her perspectives: 'How do we know whether we are learning enough?'.

CASE STUDY

The requests from the students depicted in this case scenario are commonplace. This is particularly noticeable in clinical settings where self-directed learning takes precedence over didactic modes of preclinical years.

Mentoring provides clinical teachers with a unique opportunity to follow up a group of students over a period of time. Such longitudinal follow-up allows the mentor to forge a closer relationship with students, identify their strengths and weaknesses, and support them towards advancing their studies. One of the critical supports that a mentor can provide is to guide the students in setting up their learning goals and monitoring their progress.

How do we diagnose learning problems in students?

The first step in helping a student in need of assistance is to identify the student's problem. The root cause or diagnosis for being a 'weak' student can be many including a lack of guidance, lack of motivation, poor learning techniques, personal and social issues, and psychological problems. The intervention needed for each of these problems needs to be different. Unless a mentor diagnoses the learning problem in the student with accuracy, the intervention or treatment will be misdirected.

How do we set learning goals and targets for the students?

Learning goals and targets need to be developed systematically. The process includes: (1) reviewing the curriculum goals and competencies expected of a student; (2) developing personal learning goals and targets by the students; and (3) reviewing and modifying the goals and targets set by the mentor.

How can we provide guidance to high-achieving students?

Typically in a mentoring and student monitoring system, the good students are left out. This is justifiable to some extent as there could be a resource limitation and resources need to be directed to more urgent areas, such as helping weaker students. However, high-achieving students also need attention to keep them further engaged in their learning, to direct them to areas of their interests and strengths, and to provide stress management counselling. Failure to acknowledge their unique needs may demotivate them or result in academic or social mishaps.

ACTION PLAN

- Give students the responsibility to develop their own targets so that they have greater ownership of their roles.
- Develop targets that are specific, realistic and achievable.
- Set short-term targets that are easy to achieve first, followed by more difficult ones to give students confidence.

- Set a Gantt chart for each actionable item with specific times.
- Arrange a follow-up meeting to discuss their progress.

> ### Take-home message
>
> - Learning needs are different for each learner; diagnosing their problems accurately is important.
> - A customized plan jointly developed between tutors and students is important.
> - Setting a specific, achievable target increases the chance of success.

Further reading

Harden RM, Crosby J. AMEE Guide No 20: The good teacher is more than a lecturer: the twelve roles of the teacher. *Medical Teacher* 2000; **22**: 334–47.

CHAPTER 11

Seek continually to improve your teaching skills

... good teachers are never satisfied with their teaching approaches ... they use reflection and students' feedback to identify areas in their teaching that can be further improved.

SA Azer, 2005

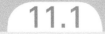

11.1

Seek to learn and incorporate new skills

Julie Quinlivan

CASE SCENARIO: LEARNING A NEW SKILL

Following a curriculum review, the head of department asked a lecturer to teach a short course in men's sexual health. The lecturer, who taught women's sexual health, felt he lacked the skills required. Furthermore, there were vocal community groups who would critically analyse the men's sexual health teaching programme.

After discussing these concerns with the head of department, the lecturer was told that he had an opportunity to acquire new skills or else have this responsibility removed; this latter option would not reflect well on the lecturer when staff were being considered for promotion.

The lecturer researched men's sexual health and identified an experienced teacher at another university and organized a meeting. At the meeting, the lecturer was told about several commercially available teaching aids, as well as the web addresses of suitable Internet sites. The experienced lecturer also suggested liaison with community groups as they could add valuable practical elements to the teaching programme. Finally, the lecturer was invited to observe classes at the other university.

The lecturer sat in on two classes and observed how the experienced lecturer managed difficult questions by referring students to resources. Community groups welcomed providing input and offered to provide a valuable practical component to the course. The lecturer acquired new teaching skills and was able to apply for promotion.

CASE STUDY

We will all eventually be asked to teach outside of our usual skill set. With increasing specialization, even specialist teachers may feel uncomfortable teaching in a subspecialty area. The strategies outlined in this scenario can be useful when a new skill set is required.

Always allocate time to learn a new skill. Most employers provide development leave or will provide time for you to acquire a new skill valuable to your organization.

Do your homework first: attend conferences and training days and read journals to learn underpinning theories. Acquire knowledge before organizing hands-on experience to maximize your gains from practical exposure.

Identify an experienced mentor through colleagues, conferences or the internet. Observing or working alongside an experienced colleague is valuable; they may be able to direct you to existing teaching resources, saving time and effort.

Liaise with community groups to see the skill set in operation.

Why is it important to acquire new skills?

It is easy to teach the same subjects every year. However, acquiring new skills leads to personal development. Spending time acquiring new skills expands your teaching repertoire.

Successful teachers are proactive and tackle the challenge of new technologies and skills.

What strategies will you use to achieve your goals?

- Allocate time to learn the new skills.
- Do your research first.
- Identify teaching resources already developed and available.
- Work alongside an experienced mentor and make the time to observe or assist them.

ACTION PLAN

To acquire new skills, consider the following actions.

- Allocate time to acquire new skills. Consider applying for development leave or schedule time in your diary.
- Do your homework first.
- Identify a mentor who has the skill set you wish to acquire.
- Use existing resources.

> ### Take-home message
>
> - Even experienced teachers need to continue to acquire new skills.

Further reading

Bowen JL, Eckstrom E, Muller M, Haney E. Enhancing the effectiveness of One-Minute Preceptor faculty development workshops. *Teaching and Learning in Medicine* 2006; **18**: 35–41.

Dennick R. Long-term retention of teaching skills after attending the Teaching Improvement Project: a longitudinal, self-evaluation study. *Medical Teacher* 2003; **25**: 314–18.

Rabatin JS, Lipkin M Jr, Rubin AS *et al.* A year of mentoring in academic medicine: case report and qualitative analysis of fifteen hours of meetings between a junior and senior faculty member. *Journal of General Internal Medicine* 2004; **19**: 569–73.

Seek feedback and criticism

Marcus A Henning

CASE SCENARIO: HOW CAN I IMPROVE

I have been asked to teach a two-hour session on professionalism to a group of third-year medical students. I began with a short session on 'what is professionalism?' and 'what it means to be professional'. The students discussed this in small groups and then we discussed their ideas as a class, after which we started to relate the notion of professionalism to clinical practise and I started to link the ideas to moral reasoning and integrity. I stated my learning outcomes at the beginning of the session and finished with a summary of the lesson.

I think and feel that this session went well. But how do I know that it went well until I seek feedback from several sources, such as students and peers?

CASE STUDY

In this case, I am trying to teach several ideas to the students related to definitions around professionalism and what it means to be professional in a general sense. Then I begin to link the idea of professionalism to clinical practise with underlying themes of moral reasoning and integrity. My first question to myself is: Have I tried to do too much in a short period of time, or conversely have I not done enough? Second, have I used too much theory? And what have the students actually learned from the session? I need to be very careful when asking for feedback to avoid getting spurious responses. For example, if I simply ask the students, 'Did you like this session?', they may say, 'yes, it was cool!'. And I go away thinking I have done a good job.

Seeking feedback

Snadden and Ker suggest that there are several elements to feedback and these include clarity, ownership, frequency, balance and specificity. Similarly, Archer sees feedback as an integrative system that needs to be considered in terms of type, structure and timing. Furthermore, Archer states that we as teachers need to develop a culture of feedback by embracing the idea of continuous reflection. In this way, we continuously look for the opportunity and means to gain profitable feedback with the intention of being and becoming better teachers. Roberts also considers some of the mechanisms that can inform teaching such as obtaining multisource feedback from self, participants, colleagues and supervisors, and collating this feedback within a portfolio.

Cultivating the culture of feedback

- Creating mechanisms for students and peers to provide constructive feedback.
- Questionnaires, interviews and focus groups are effective vessels for gaining feedback.
- Developing a culture of respect and reciprocity around the learning process is essential so that all stakeholders can learn from every teaching opportunity.
- Making sure we ask the right questions is critical, as is being prepared for answers that we may not expect.
- We need to consider the context of learning and the characteristics of the people providing the feedback. For example, students may be able to give feedback about enthusiasm and understanding, but peers may be able to provide information about content accuracy.
- We have to promote and develop a culture of feedback that is linked to our organizational goals.

ACTION PLAN

To create a culture of feedback in your organization, consider the following actions.

- Encourage an open and respectful learning environment so that students and peers feel safe about providing feedback.

- Link the idea of feedback to the notion of professionalism and lifelong learning with the intent of improving the practise of teaching and developing performance.
- Develop a series of questionnaires that are reliable and valid and fit for purpose.
- Provide a neutral environment where students and peers could engage in group or individual discussions.
- Create a provision for staff development whereby teachers can ask for assistance to meet their needs for developing further proficiency.
- Create opportunities for further development, such as providing and allocating time for up-skilling and scholarship.
- Attendance at educational conferences and workshops will engender development and keep you abreast of the latest educational techniques and theories.

Take-home message

- Teaching and learning are two sides of the same coin. To be better teachers, we need to continuously seek feedback that is clear, specific and constructive. We need to be respectful and reflective about the type of feedback we receive and have systems in place to facilitate learning from the feedback.

Further reading

Archer JC. State of the science in health professional education: effective feedback. *Medical Education* 2010; **44**: 101–8.

Roberts NK. Documenting the trajectory of your teaching. In: Jeffries WB, Huggett KN (eds). *An introduction to medical teaching.* Dordrecht: Springer, 2010.

Snadden D, Ker JS. Communication skills. In: Dent JA, Harden RM (eds). *A practical guide for the medical teacher.* Edinburgh: Elsevier Churchill Livingstone, 2005.

Keep up to date in your specialty

Samy A Azer, Mubarak bin Fahad Al-Faran and Muslim Al-Saadi

CASE SCENARIO: JUST FOR THE SAKE OF MAINTENANCE OF LICENSURE

Dr Diana Creckmore has been in general practise for over 20 years. She owns a busy medical centre and is committed to her career. Although she has attended a number of continuing medical education programmes and has registered in a number of such programmes on-line, she does not enjoy completing them. Sometimes she feels that such programmes are time-consuming and unnecessary. She completes them for the sake of maintaining her licensure. Because she is not engaged or interested in continuous learning, she has not made any changes to her daily clinical practise.

CASE STUDY

This case raises an important issue about continuing medical education and keeping up to date. Some doctors, like Dr Creckmore, may become too busy and uninterested in learning new skills or keeping up to date in their specialty. Such an attitude may be due to a number of reasons: (1) the continuing medical education (CME) programmes are instructor-centred rather than learner-centred; (2) CME programmes are not integrated with professional development; (3) CME programmes are not designed in a way that aims at performance and quality improvement; (4) CME programmes are focused on time-based learning rather than on value-based learning; and (5) CME programmes are not engaging learners and not focused on areas of need.

Why do clinical teachers need to keep up to date in the area of their specialty?

- The corpus of knowledge related to medical practise is continually progressing.
- There are constant changes in the health-care delivery and health system.
- There is increasing demand for patient safety and quality outcomes in patient safety.
- There are new medical procedures being developed that demand training before their implementation.

ACTION PLAN

To keep up to date, consider the following actions.

- Select the programmes that cover the knowledge and skills you need to acquire.
- Commit yourself to get the most out of these programmes.
- Do your homework first.
- Reflect on what you have learnt and think about strategies you will use to apply your new skills.
- Ask a mentor who has the skill you wish to acquire to assess your work and give you feedback on tasks you have completed.

Take-home message

- Clinical teachers cannot practise competently without keeping up to date in the area of their expertise.
- Active participation by giving and receiving is the optimum way for keeping up to date.

Further reading

Armstrong E, Parsa-Parsi R. How can physicians' learning styles drive educational planning? *Academic Medicine* 2005; **80**: 680–4.

Dauphinee WD. Educators must consider patient outcomes when assessing the impact of clinical training. *Medical Education* 2012; **46**: 13–20.

Dorman T, Miller BM. Continuing medical education: the link between physician learning and health care outcomes. *Academic Medicine* 2011; **86**: 1339.

Use technology to facilitate teaching and learning

Samy A Azer and Sami Al-Nassar

CASE SCENARIO

Frank Gatesman is a university professor with over 30 years of experience in anatomy. He is currently chairing the Department of Anatomy and Molecular Biology. Although he is passionate about teaching anatomy, he does not support the use of technology-based educational programmes in teaching/learning anatomy. He only believes in traditional teaching methods, such as lectures and dissection.

Two years ago, the Department of Medical Education invited him to join the e-learning and technology-based educational committee. However, it seems from the committee minutes that he is not supporting the use of e-learning or any of the newly developed technology-based educational programmes in learning anatomy. Because of his repeated failure to demonstrate leadership, particularly at the time the faculty was changing its medical curriculum, another professor was invited to chair the Department of Anatomy and Molecular Biology.

CASE STUDY

With the changes introduced in medical and allied health curricula, the use of technology-based educational programmes has become a priority. This case presents a typical example of resistance to change in implementing the use of e-learning in the curriculum. Teachers may find it difficult to support the change, particularly if they lack information and experience in the area of current educational approaches and outcomes of research in this area. Other sources of resistance may include: (1) lack of skills in developing an integrated curriculum and how to use technology-based educational programmes in the new design; (2) insufficient knowledge about the outcomes of the new curriculum; (3) not

CASE STUDY (continued)

having the resources to execute the changes in the curriculum; and (4) fear of losing control of the curriculum and its implementation. Teachers should ask the following questions prior to making a decision to introduce technology-based educational programmes.

- What do we hope to accomplish?
- Will these technology-based educational programmes allow students to more effectively and efficiently achieve the learning outcomes?
- How will these programmes engage the learner?
- What exactly will the learner do?
- How will these programmes meet the needs of each learner?
- How will these programmes work with the different components of the curriculum?
- What tools of evaluation will we use?
- Are these tools valid and reliable?

How can newly introduced technology-based educational programmes be evaluated?

- Does the new idea help learners in developing their skills in problem-solving and the application of the knowledge acquired?
- Will the new idea make learning better?
- Will the new idea help students in enhancing their learning? How can we measure this?
- What are the perceived limitations of the new idea?
- How will the new idea enable the integration of knowledge?
- What are the interactive tasks included in the programme?
- Does the new idea enable the identified learning/teaching problems to be overcome? What advantages will technology-based education bring compared to traditional methods?
- What are the desired educational outcomes?

What makes teachers become uninterested in using technology-based educational programmes?

- Lack of experience with e-learning and technology-based education.
- Not interested in learning new skills.

- Not aware of the literature and new innovations in this area.
- Believe that traditional teaching is the best way to teach students.
- Not accepting change or being open to the idea of student-centred learning.
- Have limited teaching/learning skills.

ACTION PLAN

To ensure the use of technologies in facilitating teaching and learning, you may explore the following recommendations.

- Assess the educational needs of your students and how the use of e-learning and technology-based educational programmes can help in addressing these needs.
- Estimate the costs and benefits of introducing e-learning and technology-based educational programmes.
- Plan how to link e-learning and technology-based educational programmes to the design of the curriculum and self-directed learning sessions.
- Evaluate the impact of using e-learning and technology-based educational programmes on students' learning and achieving curriculum outcomes.

Take-home message

- The use of e-learning should aim at enhancing cognitive skills and application of knowledge learnt.
- Teachers should seek training in the area of e-learning, simulation, and how to use such programmes to support the curriculum.
- Evaluating the impact of e-learning and the use of technology-based learning on students' learning will help teachers in assessing the value of such programmes in achieving specific learning outcomes.

Further reading

Dror I, Schmidt P, O'Connor L. A cognitive perspective on technology enhanced learning in medical training: great opportunities, pitfalls, and challenges. *Medical Teacher* 2011; **33**: 291–6.

Issenberg SB, Gordon MS, Gordon DL *et al.* Simulation and new learning technologies. *Medical Teacher* 2001; **23**: 16–23.

McGee JB, Begg M. What medical educators need to know about web 2.0. *Medical Teacher* 2008; **30**: 164–9.

McGee JB, Kanter SL. How we develop and sustain innovation in medical education technology: keys to success. *Medical Teacher* 2011; **33**: 279–85.

Monitor your progress

Onishi Hirotaka

CASE SCENARIO: IS MY TEACHING OK?

Three years have passed since Dr Sato, one of the preceptors in a general internal medicine ward, finished his postgraduate specialty training. He taught in rounds/conferences every day and tried hard to deliver clinical knowledge to medical students in a mini-lecture format, but their tiresome attitude annoyed him very much. The clinical teaching director asked him to attend a faculty development workshop in an annual national conference for medical education. He learned two things in the workshop. (1) Effective questioning is more beneficial for medical students to actively think about clinical medicine than mini-lectures, and (2) five-step microskills are useful for effective questioning.

He was satisfied with the usefulness of two important questions: 'What do you think differential diagnoses are?' and 'Why do you think so?' for five-step microskills, but he was not confident about how he should give students feedback. 'Is my teaching skill OK for students?' He felt more anxious about his teaching than before.

CASE STUDY

This scenario describes how clinical teachers improve their teaching. Normally, a few years after the completion of postgraduate training, clinical teachers become competent in clinical practise, but not in clinical teaching. Some clinical teachers do not know what they do not know, or what they can't do to achieve good teaching. Staff development workshops are excellent opportunities to understand their own weaknesses in teaching.

What did he learn in the workshop?

In this case, Dr Sato learned not only the hands-on teaching model of five-step microskills, but also strengths of active involvement of clinical teachers for teaching, such as asking questions. Furthermore, he understood that how he teaches is as important as what he should teach. Soon after he learned of the technique, he started to implement it. He found a need for the specific steps of the five-step microskills and the importance of monitoring his improvement in teaching.

How can he monitor the progress of his teaching?

First, he should ask the students if they understand the clinical content in an appropriate way. An informal dialogue is usually sufficient to establish whether the students have accepted and understood what the clinical teacher would like students to learn. If the undergraduate clinical education system uses a questionnaire for teacher evaluation, such official data can be used for monitoring the progress of teaching.

Reflection as self-monitoring of teaching methods

In 1983, Schön stated that reflective practise is 'the capacity to reflect on an action so as to engage in a process of continuous learning' and 'one of the defining characteristics of professional practise'. Since both clinicians and educators improve by reflective practise, this theory is also applicable to clinical educators. Newly learned teaching skills in the workshop seemed to stimulate Dr Sato's reflective practise of clinical teaching.

Mentoring

For continuous professional development, the existence of a mentor is valuable. In this case, the clinical teaching director knew Dr Sato's teaching level and in what ways the workshop helped Dr Sato improve his teaching. In the future, whenever Dr Sato feels anxious about his teaching, he can discuss what he should do with his director and will be guided along the correct path.

ACTION PLAN

To start monitoring the progress of your teaching, consider the following actions.

- Critically reflect on your own teaching. If you do not have knowledge/skills to reflect on your teaching, consider attending staff development activities.

- Ask if students are satisfied with your teaching for the purpose of monitoring.

- Find a mentor for your continuous professional development.

> ### Take-home message
>
> - It will take a long time for you to become an excellent clinical teacher. However, a journey of a thousand miles begins with a single step.

Further reading

Neher JO, Gordon KG, Meyer B, Stevens N. A five-step 'microskill' model of clinical teaching. *Journal of the American Board of Family Physicians* 1992; **5**: 419–23.

Schön, D. *The reflective practitioner: how professionals think in action.* New York: Basic Books, 1983.

Spencer J. ABC of learning and teaching in medicine – learning and teaching in the clinical environment. *British Medical Journal* 2003; **326**: 591–4.

CHAPTER 12

Demonstrate leadership in teaching

*Becoming an excellent leader begins with a basic
understanding of what leadership is and how these skills can
best be developed … skills needed to be an effective leader are
dynamic and constantly changing in response to a rapidly
changing world.*

J-A Sawatzky *et al.*, 2009

12.1	Contribute to course design and structure
12.2	Contribute to publications on education
12.3	Demonstrate self-development in an educational context
12.4	Demonstrate creativity in teaching strategies
12.5	Be committed to professional development
12.6	Share in managing changes in curriculum and educational needs

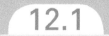

Contribute to course design and structure

Ian Wilson

CASE SCENARIO: I PUT A GREAT DEAL OF WORK INTO IT

Michael is a newly qualified consultant who has recently started in a position in a teaching hospital. Shortly after starting, he was invited to join a group of hospital doctors who were planning the implementation of a new curriculum for medical students working in the hospital. At the second group meeting, he was asked if he could prepare a series of three tutorials introducing the students to the management of the patient with headaches. This was a topic he knew well, and he quickly agreed.

In thinking about how to teach this topic, he remembered his teaching as very dry and piecemeal. He was determined to make the tutorials very clinical and to lead the students through mechanisms, diagnosis and management. Michael spent many hours putting together a polished programme that took the student from no knowledge through to a detailed understanding of the pathophysiology of headaches and then to diagnosis of management. He was quietly confident it would be a success.

Fourteen of the possible 15 students arrived for the first tutorial and it started enthusiastically, but the students soon looked bored and 10 minutes into the tutorial Michael was asked if the students were going to be examined on this material. He did not know the answer to this and said so. The second tutorial was even worse with only four students attending and the last tutorial was not attended by any students.

In discussing this with a colleague, he discovered that the students were in their final few months of the course, not just starting as he had thought, and the material was definitely assessable. Michael learned that a large amount of work does not necessarily result in success.

CASE STUDY

There are a number of issues in this scenario where, despite a significant effort, Michael was not able to deliver a programme that benefited the students. The most obvious issue for Michael was not being aware of the students' prior level of knowledge. The lack of knowledge can lead to going over old material or starting way beyond where the students are. The second issue relates to assessment. A common aphorism is that 'assessment drives learning'. While this has not been specifically researched it has been well demonstrated that assessment has a significant impact on learning.

Why is it important to be involved in course design and structure?

Educational experts could have provided Michael with advice that might have helped prevent his problems, but they cannot provide the clinical or scientific input that the students require. Clinicians are essential to the development of curriculum for clinical topics. Understanding a few basic principles will enable a clinician to develop and implement educational programmes that appeal to students.

What strategies will you use to achieve your goals?

- Determine the students' prior knowledge – are they beginners or experienced?
- Determine what you want the students to be able to demonstrate after the course. This is known as developing learning outcomes.
- Based on your learning outcomes, devise your assessment. If you are to teach students about lumbar puncture your assessment will depend if you want them to demonstrate knowledge of the principles of performing a lumbar puncture or that they can demonstrate competence in the procedure. For principles, your assessment could be written papers, while to demonstrate, you may use simulation.
- Based on your assessment, determine your method of teaching. Principles could be taught in a lecture or tutorial, while undertaking the procedure may require a simulation centre.

ACTION PLAN

To ensure that you take part in curriculum development and implementation:

- Learn a few basic educational principles
- Seek the advice of educational experts if necessary
- Remember you are the content expert.

Take-home message

- To contribute to course design and structure, learn a few basic educational principles.
- Learn how to write learning outcomes.

Further reading

Amin Z, Khoo HE. *Basics in medical education*. Singapore: World Scientific Publishing, 2003.

Contribute to publications on education

Ian Wilson

CASE SCENARIO: WHY WON'T THEY PUBLISH IT?

A general practitioner working in conjunction with a training programme was asked to develop an educational module for the trainees. The module was developed and implemented and the resultant evaluation was excellent. The trainees all enjoyed the module and felt their knowledge and skills were now better than when they started. The director of the training programme was impressed with the results and recommended that the module be published.

The general practitioner wrote up the module and submitted it to a journal. It was rejected by the editor shortly after as it was not submitted in the manner required by the journal. The editor suggested accessing the author instructions on the website. After reading the author instructions and painstakingly changing the references and reformatting, the paper was resubmitted. It was rejected again as it did not fit with the style used by the journal. After looking at other journals and the author instructions, it was rewritten and submitted to a second journal. This time it was accepted by the editor and referred to two referees.

Six long weeks later, a response was received from the editor and referees – rejection. The reviewers highlighted a number of issues, most correctable, but two that could not be corrected. The first was that ethics approval had not been obtained for the study. In a large number of countries, this is now a requirement. Second, the reviewers did not accept positive attitudes and self-perceived changes from the participants as demonstrating the educational success of the module.

One year later, the module was repeated with prior ethics approval for the collection of data and a pre- and post-knowledge test undertaken and the result was published by the journal.

CASE STUDY

The scenario describes a not uncommon set of issues that befall the novice author. It is not their educational intervention that is the problem, but the mechanics of getting published. It is not uncommon for someone to develop a module and at the end feel that it was so successful that it needs to be published. It is then that the problems start. The mechanics of submitting papers is complicated and specific to each journal. Formatting requirements vary and referencing systems are different and even the method of submission varies between journals.

Why is it important to be involved in publishing papers?

It is vitally important that innovations in education are published so that the methods are taken up (and improved) by others. This may save others time and provide them with evidence of success.

What strategies will you use to achieve your goals?

- When devising an educational programme, consider whether to publish the results or not.
- If ethics are an issue, make sure you have ethics approval prior to collecting any data.
- Make sure the data you collect indicate a change in knowledge, performance or attitudes and devise your data collection appropriately.
- Read the author instructions carefully and follow them explicitly before submitting your paper.
- Use a referencing system so that changes to the format of the references can be managed easily.
- Seek the help of someone who has publishing experience to help you navigate the system.

ACTION PLAN

To ensure that you take part in publishing:

- Think about publishing while developing or improving your programmes
- Seek the advice of someone experienced in having their work published
- Take the time to assess the success of your programme in a form that is publishable.

Take-home message

- For the benefit of other teachers and students, publish your innovative education programmes.
- Have a mentor help you navigate the publishing process the first time you publish.

Further reading

Association for the Study of Medical Education. *The clinical teacher.* Blackwell Publishing. Available from: www.theclinicalteacher.com.

Association for the Study of Medical Education. Really good stuff. Published annually in *Medical Education* by Wiley Blackwell. Available from: www.mededuc.com.

Demonstrate self-development in an educational context

Chi-Wan Lai

CASE SCENARIO: GETTING STUDENTS TO BE MORE ENGAGED IN BEDSIDE TEACHING

A faculty member who had been very dedicated to clinical teaching at the bedside confessed to his colleague that even though he had tried to teach not only medical knowledge, clinical and communication skills, but also attitude in terms of treating patients with respect, he was discouraged by the students' responses. His colleague advised him to ask his students why they could not respond to his teaching with the same enthusiasm as him, and what he could do to engage them more.

The students responded, 'We don't see how your teaching is relevant with respect to our need of becoming better physicians'. The teacher thought about it, searched for pertinent literature on the subject, and modified his teaching. He attended workshops offered by his institution's Centre for Faculty Development, and cultivated the habit of constantly jotting down ideas he came across for improvement. His students responded enthusiastically to his teachings later on.

CASE STUDY

Clinical teaching at the bedside is challenging because the content of the teaching depends almost exclusively on the case being presented, and the teacher has to switch back and forth from a mode of patient-centred care to learner-centred teaching during ward rounds. To make clinical teaching interesting to students, teachers have to make the contents relevant, engage the students and adapt the teaching methods accordingly. They have to learn how to teach effectively and improve themselves continuously. To do so, they have to know what skills a good teacher should acquire first.

What competencies do medical educators require?

Scholars have listed the various roles teachers play, or the core qualities they should possess, but a helpful conceptual model is the framework of teaching competencies developed by Srinivasan and colleagues based on the ACGME framework. The six core competencies of medical educators are: medical (or content) knowledge, learner-centredness, interpersonal and communication skills, professionalism and role-modelling, practise-based reflection, and systems-based practise. Educators with programmatic roles have four additional specialized competencies: program design/implementation, evaluation/scholarship, leadership and mentorship. Many of these skills can be learnt by oneself, and of the various skills for self-development, scholars have particularly advocated self-reflection.

How to engage in self-reflection on teaching?

Self-reflection involves analysing, questioning, reframing and assessing an experience in order for one to learn from it and to improve practise. Although clinicians have very busy schedules, they can still conduct self-reflection by simply jotting down notes about their own observations and ideas on particular issues. They can also analyse special events or critical incidents, or think through a particular problem. The best method, however, is using a journal to critically examine one's underlying assumptions and the impact of one's actions, gain a different perspective, build self-awareness, and derive means of improving one's future actions. One can check the depth of one's writing by analysing the different levels of reflection in one's journal, from reporting, responding, relating and reasoning through to reconstructing.

ACTION PLAN

Strategies for improving teaching and developing the self in education:

- Soliciting feedback from students
- Engaging in self-reflection
- Keeping up to date with the literature
- Attending workshops on faculty development

- Using videotaping and role play to improve teaching
- Participating in a peer group, or having 'critical friends' to obtain feedback and critique
- Being mentored by a more senior physician
- Engaging in educational scholarship.

Take-home message

- Self-development in education is a continuous process, and can be achieved through self-reflection, soliciting feedback from peers, students and mentors, or through the use of technology, such as videotaping, and keeping abreast of new teaching and learning.
- Self-reflection is a good method to improve one's self and teaching, and it can be done by cultivating awareness, analysing one's experiences or through journal writing.

Further reading

Aronson L. Twelve tips for teaching reflection at all levels of medical education. *Medical Teacher* 2011; **33**: 200–5.

McLean M, Cilliers F, Van Wyk JM. Faculty development: yesterday, today and tomorrow. *Medical Teacher* 2008; **30**: 555–84.

Srinivasan M, Li ST, Pratt DD *et al.* 'Teaching as a competency': competencies for medical educators. *Academic Medicine* 2011; **86**: 1211–20.

Demonstrate creativity in teaching strategies

Julie Quinlivan

CASE SCENARIO: DEMONSTRATE CREATIVITY IN TEACHING

The curriculum included learning outcomes for clinical ultrasound examination. Learning resources were provided in the form of five lectures, two written case-based small group tutorials and a problem-based learning (PBL) case. Students were rostered to attend two hospital ultrasound clinics.

Assessment analysis demonstrated that students performed well in theoretical outcomes, but poorly in practical and applied tasks. Student evaluation indicated that they had poor access to clinical learning resources.

It was decided to review the learning resources. The cost of delivering the existing programme was calculated to generate a budget.

Staff agreed to implement a cost equivalent set of innovative learning resources which involved two theoretical lectures, each followed by practical small group tutorials where students performed ultrasounds on donated machines utilizing commercial models able to demonstrate ultrasound features of blood in the abdominal cavity, breech presentation, gallstones and musculoskeletal haematoma. There were a further four on-line cases with images and an on-line resource for students to complete as self-directed learning activities. Students still attended two clinics.

Assessment analysis demonstrated high levels of both theoretical and practical understanding of learning outcomes and the practical tutorials were rated highly as a learning resource in student evaluation.

CASE STUDY

Analysis of assessment data by learning outcome is a useful method to identify problem areas in curriculum delivery. When poor results are achieved in a domain, review and change are important. In clinical teaching, students are motivated and clever, so poor outcomes at a year level suggest a problem with the resources available to facilitate student learning. In this case, students achieved theoretical outcomes, but were deficient in clinical and applied tasks.

As access to clinical patients becomes limited, the use of models and simulation has increased. In developing countries, there are usually sufficient patients in clinical settings for workplace-based learning and the argument for 'simulated' learning resources is difficult to justify. In contrast, in developed countries, students may compete for clinical resources.

Companies and hospitals are often willing to donate second-hand equipment to establish low-cost simulation. There are many commercially available models for teaching. This enables students to be accredited in skills in a simulated environment before accessing patients.

Creativity can also be applied to theoretical learning outcomes through interprofessional education, team-based problem solving and on-line learning programmes. PBL, considered innovative, is now 25 years old, and many variants exist.

Creativity in teaching also extends to assessment with focus increasingly on assessment measuring applied knowledge rather than factual recall, achieved through integrated assessment tasks, script concordance testing and 360° workplace-based assessments.

Why is it important to demonstrate creativity?

- Creative approaches can help when learning outcomes are poor and need revision.
- Improvements in technology can help overcome limited access to patients.
- Innovation in teaching needs to be matched with innovation in assessment measuring higher-order outcomes involving application of knowledge.

What strategies will you use to achieve your goals?

- Innovation requires effort, so it is best to use your energy in areas where learning outcomes are suboptimal.
- Other staff need to support the concept of change and departmental heads will want change to be cost neutral, so budgeting is vital.
- Look at the research literature for innovative ideas that address your areas of poor performance.
- Remember that innovation can cover both teaching and assessment modalities.

ACTION PLAN

To achieve innovation, consider the following actions.

- Identify areas where learning outcomes are suboptimal.
- Agree to an innovative cost-neutral change with colleagues.
- Attend conferences for ideas.
- Read medical education journals.
- Match innovation in teaching with innovation in assessment.

Take-home message

- Focus innovation in areas where teaching outcomes are poor.

Further reading

Cauraugh JH, Martin M, Martin KK. Modeling surgical expertise for motor skill acquisition. *American Journal of Surgery* 1999; **177**: 331–6.

Perciful EG, Nester PA. The effect of an innovative clinical teaching method on nursing students' knowledge and critical thinking skills. *Journal of Nursing Education* 1996; **35**: 23–8.

Womack B, Hall A. Innovative clinical teaching. *Advanced Clinical Care* 1991; **6**: 26–7.

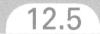

Be committed to professional development

Sam Leinster

CASE SCENARIO: A CONCERNED DEAN

The dean was very concerned about teaching in the Department of Surgery. The members of faculty in the department were conscientious in delivering teaching, but the student evaluation of the quality of the teaching had fallen for the third year in succession. The dean called a meeting with the senior members of the department to discuss the problem. At the meeting it became clear that the faculty had high levels of engaging in continuing professional development (CPD) for their clinical roles. They held regular departmental review meetings and journal clubs. Members of the department regularly attended national and international scientific meetings and reported the information gained back to their colleagues. None had ever attended a CPD event relating to learning and teaching. They were not aware of the findings of the student evaluation although the results had been sent regularly to the department head. When asked how they planned their teaching, they stated that they copied what they had experienced as students.

CASE STUDY

Continuous quality improvement is an important component of all professional activities. Reflection and self-awareness are essential prerequisites for such improvement. As an individual or a team reflects on their performance, they will become aware of areas where performance could be improved. Ideally, this will be followed by a more detailed examination of the situation leading to an exact diagnosis of the problem and a plan for correcting it. Where the diagnosis includes learning needs (deeper knowledge or new skills), the plan will include an appropriate learning plan.

CASE STUDY

The Department of Surgery in the example appear to behave appropriately in this regard with respect to their clinical practise. However, they display a not uncommon attitude that teaching is an intuitive activity that has not changed over time. As a result, they do not see any need to review their teaching practise or develop their educational skills. Within the clinical area, they accept that knowledge is constantly changing and that new skills need to be mastered. They are unaware that education is also a constantly developing field.

Educational development should be treated in the same way as other professional development. Self-review is mandatory and this is greatly facilitated if it incorporates input from colleagues. A peer-mentoring arrangement with another teacher can be helpful. If a department wishes to provide a consistently high standard of education, it should hold regular meetings at which the educational activities are reviewed. This, of course, includes a formal review of the results of any evaluations that have taken place. Some mechanism for keeping up to date with developments in education should be set up, including attendance by at least some of the members of the department at relevant meetings and workshops. Any appraisal system that is set up should include appraisal of teaching and make appropriate plans for professional development in this area.

ACTION PLAN

- Undertake regular reflection on your personal performance as a teacher.
- Find a mentor – this can be a more senior colleague or a peer whom you respect.
- Read journals on medical education – these may come free with membership of a relevant learned society.
- Set up a regular meeting to review educational activities and discuss educational developments.
- Attend national and international meetings and workshops on education.

> ## Take-home message
>
> - Teaching is a professional activity which should be approached with the same attitude to continuous quality improvement as other professional activities.

Further reading

Davis N, Davis D, Bloch R. Continuing medical education – AMEE Guide 35. *Medical Teacher* 2008; **30**: 652–66.

Schön D. *Educating the reflective practitioner: toward a new design for teaching and learning in the professions.* San Francisco: Jossey-Bass, 1987.

Share in managing changes in curriculum and educational needs

Mohammad Y Al-Shehri and Samy A Azer

CASE SCENARIO: DOES NOT BELIEVE IN CURRICULUM CHANGE

Roxana Malki has been an academic in a major university for over 15 years. However, she does not believe in curriculum change and the new strategies available, such as problem-based learning, small group discussion and integration across disciplines. She feels that such changes will not benefit basic sciences and will not enhance the teaching and learning of these sciences.

Because of these beliefs, Roxana was critical about the new curriculum introduced in her school. Although she attended training workshops about the facilitation of problem-based learning cases in tutorials, she did not facilitate the group discussion, but rather gave her students a lecture about the case. Her attitude and negative statements were not beneficial to the successful delivery of the curriculum and caused a number of students to face challenges in effectively understanding the material.

CASE STUDY

This case scenario shows how teachers' viewpoints about curriculum design could affect their behaviour and performance during the process of curriculum implementation. The Department of Medical Education and those leading the process of curriculum management should be aware of such challenges and be prepared to handle such situations. Staff training may help in enhancing teachers' facilitation skills and prepare them for curriculum change. However, not all teachers will benefit from such training programmes. As outlined in this scenario, Roxana

CASE STUDY (continued)

has declared her opposition to the process of curriculum change. Despite her comments and views, she participated in faculty training programmes and became a PBL tutor. It appears that the training programme did not help her in changing her views about the new curriculum and her role as group facilitator. To help teachers become active participants in curriculum change and curriculum management, the Department of Medical Education should endorse faculty training programmes that: (1) enable staff monitoring and learning through constructive feedback; (2) help teachers develop skills in curriculum management and successful implementation; and (3) allow teachers to not just change their views but become active participants in curriculum management and successful implementation.

Why do medical and allied health schools change their curricula?

The rationale for curriculum change may include:

- Providing a high standard of patient-centred care
- Ensuring that graduates are able to implement the 'best practise' approach in their career
- Providing students with tools for continuing improvement of their learning
- Ensuring that students have developed competencies and skills needed for their career
- Ensuring that graduates have developed effective communication skills and are able to complete tasks professionally.

How can teachers contribute to the management of curriculum change?

- Work collaboratively with the Department of Medical Education.
- Take an active role in the management of curriculum delivery.
- Provide constructive feedback to the Department of Medical Education.

ACTION PLAN

- The Department of Medical Education has a responsibility to engage clinical teachers in the different aspects of curriculum change.

- Preparation of the faculty for change is vital and should start three to four years prior to the implementation of the new curriculum.

- Teachers should be clear about their roles and responsibilities.

- Teachers can share by their active participation in the implementation of the new curriculum. Examples of these roles include chairing a block/module, becoming a PBL tutor, participating in the committees responsible for writing PBL cases, and participating in the assessment and evaluation task groups.

Take-home message

- Although the management of curriculum delivery is the responsibility of the Department of Medical Education, all teachers have a role in ensuring its successful delivery.

- The support of teachers for the process of curriculum change enhances successful delivery and achieving optimum outcomes.

- The changes associated with the introduction of a patient-centred, integrated curriculum could result in a cultural shift toward relationship-centredness within the institution.

Further reading

Azer SA. Introducing a problem-based learning program: 12 tips for success. *Medical Teacher* 2011; **33**: 808–13.

Christianson CE, McBride RB, Vari RC *et al*. From traditional to patient-centered learning: curriculum change as an intervention for changing institutional culture and promoting professionalism in undergraduate medical education. *Academic Medicine* 2007; **82**: 1079–88.

Schwartz PL, Loten EG, Miller AP. Curriculum reform at the University of Otago Medical School. *Academic Medicine* 1999; **74**: 675–9.

CHAPTER 13

Contribute to and appreciate the value of research

Scholarship as applied to academic life is generally understood to mean the creation of new knowledge and its dissemination through peer review and publication.

SP Mennin and MC McGrew, 2000

13.1

Use evidence-based teaching in enhancing clinical teaching skills

Samy A Azer

CASE SCENARIO: I DO NOT BELIEVE IN THE NEW WAYS OF TEACHING

Robert Angus is a clinical teacher with over 20 years of experience in patient care and teaching. He feels that his main commitment should be directed to patient care. Although he has contributed to clinical teaching for several years, he believes that his job as a teacher is to provide students with knowledge and skills. However, his sessions lack interaction with students and do not allow students to think, work on tasks, develop their clinical skills or receive feedback. He always thought that his teaching sessions suit the needs of his students and he should not make any changes to his teaching style. Yesterday, and for the first time in his career, he attended a training workshop on clinical teaching. He was shocked by the initiatives discussed in the workshop sessions regarding active learning and evidence-based teaching.

CASE STUDY

This case scenario highlights the state of a good number of teachers who lack knowledge and skills in facilitation, active learning and teaching strategies that could adequately prepare them in their teaching. The scenario also raises the need for teachers to develop their teaching skills and make their sessions student-centred, with an emphasis on professionalism, competency-based assessment and clinical skills.

What are the common challenges observed in clinical teaching sessions?

In 2003, John Spencer identified a number of common challenges in clinical teaching. Examples of these challenges include:

- Lack of active participation of learners
- Sessions focused on factual knowledge, rather than problem solving
- Lack of clear objectives for sessions
- Inadequate feedback provided to the learners
- Lack of alignment with the rest of the curriculum.

How can clinical teachers enhance their teaching skills and what are the teaching/learning strategies they could include in their teaching?

Continuous training in clinical teaching and how to implement new teaching strategies is vital. Teaching strategies that can enhance clinical teaching include:

- Creating an environment that enables learners to feel safe, discuss their views and make comments
- Teaching students how to apply knowledge learnt from one patient to solve new problems
- Reinforcing what was learnt and was done well by students
- Providing constructive feedback and allowing students to learn from their mistakes.

ACTION PLAN

To use evidence-based teaching in enhancing clinical teaching skills, the following steps may be of value.

- Continuous training of teachers in training programmes that aim at enhancing teaching skills and current principles of teaching is essential.
- Clinical teachers' reflection on their teaching role helps to reinforce their role and enables them to seek training.
- Clinical teachers have to readjust their teaching approaches to match with the changes introduced in the curriculum, and base their teaching on evidence from education research and current practises.

> ## Take-home message
>
> - Clinical teachers have a responsibility to receive appropriate training in clinical teaching and update their teaching skills.
> - Faculty development is a great opportunity for clinical teachers to actively participate and learn to practise evidence-based teaching.

Further reading

Neale AV, Schwartz KL, Schenk MJ, Roth LM. Scholarly development of clinician faculty using evidence-based medicine as an organizing theme. *Medical Teacher* 2003; **25**: 442–7.

Pitkäla K, Mäntyranta T, Strandberg TE *et al.* Evidence-based medicine – how to teach critical science thinking to medical undergraduates. *Medical Teacher* 2000; **22**: 22–6.

Ramani S, Leinster S. AMEE guide no 34: Teaching in the clinical environment. *Medical Teacher* 2008; **30**: 347–64.

Spencer J. Learning and teaching in the clinical environment. *British Medical Journal* 2003; **15**: 591–4.

Contribute to research in clinical education

Samy A Azer

CASE SCENARIO: HOW CAN I START?

Lydia Goodman is a general internist with over 23 years' experience in patient care. Although she has some interest in medical education, she never thought about the need to work on research projects related to medical education. This year, she attended an international conference on medical education and thoroughly enjoyed contributing to the discussion in the sessions she attended. The conference kept her motivated and triggered a number of ideas that she wanted to explore in her school. However, she was faced with the challenge of how she could go about starting a small group in her school that was interested in working with her on a medical education research project.

CASE STUDY

In this case, the clinical teacher was new to medical education research. Although she has been teaching for a long time, she never realized the need to contribute to research in medical education. A number of factors could have contributed to this deficiency. For example, she may not have realized the importance of medical education research or perhaps she was too busy attending to patient care. Other possible contributing factors may be her lack of experience or there were no groups in her school interested in medical education research that she can join. Attending conferences on medical education is a great opportunity to learn, share and become motivated to explore new ideas and initiate research projects.

What are the challenges facing researchers interested in conducting research in medical education?

- Inadequate resources and funding.
- No recognition of research in medical education.
- Research in medical education is different from basic and clinical research.
- Lack of experience in medical education research.
- Prestigious international journals focusing on medical education research are very few and the competition to publish in them is great.

ACTION PLAN

The following actions may help clinical educators new to research in medical education.

- Dedicate time to medical education research.
- Identify barriers in your schools to conducting a scholarly project on medical education and think about strategic plans to overcome these challenges.
- Establish a small group of individuals in your school who share a passion for medical education research.
- Attend and plan to contribute to conferences on medical education in your country and other international conferences, such as the annual conference for the Association of Medical Education in Europe (AMEE).
- Work on focusing your work to reflect scholarly outcomes.

Take-home message

- Clinical educators have great opportunities and rich material for research.
- Joining a group of clinicians with interest in medical education research could help in the development of an on-going activity related to research in medical education.

Further reading

Beckman TJ, Lee MC, Ficalora RD. Experience with a medical education research group at the Mayo Clinic. *Medical Teacher* 2009; **31**: 518–21.

Carline JD. Funding medical education research: opportunities and issues. *Academic Medicine* 2004; **79**: 918–24.

Irby DM, Hodgson CS, Muller JH. Promoting research in medical education at the University of California San Francisco School of Medicine. *Academic Medicine* 2004; **79**: 981–4.

Mennin SP, Cole McGrew M. Scholarship in teaching and best evidence medical education: synergy for teaching and learning. *Medical Teacher* 2000; **22**: 468–71.

Encourage students to undertake research and publish their work

Samy A Azer

CASE SCENARIO: A BUSY SUPERVISOR

Rana, Heba and Sarah are undertaking a research project during their third medical year. Their supervisor is the head of one of the departments in the College of Medicine. During the first two weeks of commencing their research project, they are very happy as their supervisor is an influential academic in the college and devoted some of his time to them. However, over the next few weeks, they come to realize that their supervisor is always busy and does not provide them with the supervision they need. He always sends his apologies for missing meetings with them and when he meets with them, he looks distracted and unable to provide them with clear guidance or help to overcome the challenges they are facing. Their progress on the project has slowed and they feel that they will not be able to submit their research report on time.

CASE STUDY

This case highlights the importance of the role of a research supervisor in motivating students, guiding them and ensuring their consistent progress. Busy supervisors and those who do not devote quality time to their students and work effectively with them will not be able to help their students achieve their potential.

What are the benefits of enabling undergraduate students to conduct research?

Conducting research enables students to:

- Understand and be aware of the importance of research in professional development
- Become confident in their research skills

- Read and understand research papers
- Develop an interest in undertaking research degrees (e.g. Master's by research and PhDs).

What are the responsibilities of research supervisors?

- Help students in organizing and planning their time schedule for the different stages of the project.
- Facilitate the process of defining their research questions, generating their hypotheses, choosing their research methodology, interpreting their findings and discussing them in light of the current literature.
- Support students to progress and motivate them to complete their work and turn their work into an engaging experience.
- Encourage students to publish their findings.

ACTION PLAN

To encourage students to undertake research and publish their work, teachers should:

- Commit themselves to their role as research supervisors
- Work effectively with their students at the different stages of the project
- Motivate their students and help them by providing constructive feedback to successfully complete each stage in the research project as planned
- Encourage them to take the lead and work collaboratively as a team, if the research projects are allocated to groups of three or four students.

Take-home message

- Participation of undergraduate students in hands-on research enables students to experience the role of research in the advancement of medical and health professions.
- Training teachers in supervising students conducting research is vital in achieving optimum outcomes.

Further reading

Russell SH, Hancock MP, McCullough J. Benefits of undergraduate research experiences. *Science* 2007; **316**: 548–9.

Index